Biological Effects of Ultrasound

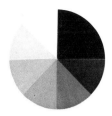

CLINICS IN DIAGNOSTIC ULTRASOUND
VOLUME 16

Volumes Already Published

Forthcoming Volumes in the Series

Biological Effects of Ultrasound

Edited by

Wesley L. Nyborg, Ph.D.

Professor of Physics
The University of Vermont
Burlington, Vermont

and

Marvin C. Ziskin, M.D., M.S. Bm.E.

Professor of Radiology and Medical Physics
Department of Diagnostic Imaging
Temple University School of Medicine
Philadelphia, Pennsylvania

CHURCHILL LIVINGSTONE
NEW YORK, EDINBURGH, LONDON, AND MELBOURNE
1985

Acquisitions editor: William R. Schmitt
Copy editor: Kim Loretucci
Production editor: Charlie Lebeda
Production supervisor: Sharon Tuder
Compositor: Kingsport Press
Printer/Binder: The Maple-Vail Book Manufacturing Group

Distributed in the United Kingdom by Churchill Livingstone, Robert Stevenson House, 1–3 Baxter's Place, Leith Walk, Edinburgh EH1 3AF and by associated companies, branches and representatives throughout the world.

First published 1985

Printed in USA

ISBN 0–443–08314–2

7 6 5 4 3 2 1

Library of Congress Cataloging in Publication Data
Main entry under title:

Biological effects of ultrasound.

   Includes bibliographies and index.
   1. Ultrasonic waves—Physiological effect.
2. Ultrasonics in medicine.   I. Nyborg, Wesley Le Mars.
II. Ziskin, Marvin C.   [DNLM: 1. Ultrasonics—adverse effects.   2. Ultrasonics—diagnostic use.
W1 CL831BC v.16 / WB 289 B615]
QP82.2.U37B56 1985   574.19'145   84–23245
ISBN 0–443–08314–2

Manufactured in the United States of America

Contributors

Edwin L. Carstensen, Ph.D.
Professor of Electrical Engineering and of Radiation Biology and Biophysics, The University of Rochester, Rochester, New York

Mary Dyson, Ph.D.
Senior Lecturer in Anatomy, Guy's Hospital Medical and Dental Schools, London, England

Allen H. Gates, Ph.D.
Assistant Professor of Radiation Biology and Biophysics (Toxicology), of Obstetrics and Gynecology, and of Genetics, The University of Rochester School of Medicine and Dentistry, Rochester, New York

Charles W. Hohler, M.D.
Director, Perinatology and Perinatal Ultrasound, St. Joseph's Hospital and Medical Center, Phoenix, Arizona

Frederick W. Kremkau, Ph.D.
Associate Professor of Diagnostic Ultrasound, Yale University School of Medicine, New Haven, Connecticut

Padmakar P. Lele, M.D., D.Phil.
Professor of Experimental Medicine, Harvard-Massachusetts Institute of Technology Division of Health Science and Technology; Director, Hyperthermia Center, Massachusetts Institute of Technology, Cambridge, Massachusetts

Morton W. Miller, Ph.D.
Senior Scientist, Associate Professor of Radiation Biology and Biophysics, The University of Rochester School of Medicine and Dentistry, Rochester, New York

Wesley L. Nyborg, Ph.D.
Professor of Physics, The University of Vermont, Burlington, Vermont

William D. O'Brien, Jr., Ph.D.
Associate Professor of Electrical and Computer Engineering and of Bioengineering, Bioacoustics Research Laboratory, University of Illinois, Urbana, Illinois

John Thacker, Ph.D.
Chairman, Cell and Molecular Biology Division, Medical Research Council Radiobiology Unit, Harwell, Didcot, Oxon, England

Peter N.T. Wells, D.Sc.
Chief Physicist, Department of Medical Physics, Bristol General Hospital, Bristol, England

A.R. Williams, Ph.D.
Senior Lecturer in Medical Biophysics, University of Manchester, Manchester, England

Marvin C. Ziskin, M.D., M.S. Bm.E.
Professor of Radiology and Medical Physics, Department of Diagnostic Imaging, Temple University School of Medicine, Philadelphia, Pennsylvania

Contents

Foreword

From time to time, the Clinics in Diagnostic Ultrasound series seeks to bring to the attention of its readers nonclinical information that is germane to our practice. This volume on the bioeffects of ultrasound is essential reading for all of us involved in clinical scanning. Although it may not be read with the same compulsive delight as many of the clinical volumes are, we all appreciate the need and value of the information contained herein. Three authoritative reports have recently been published on the bioeffects of ultrasound, but, unfortunately, these are highly technical and will most likely be read by very few clinical practitioners. For this reason, I asked two authorities in the field to provide a more digestible version to help us in our clinical practice. They have succeeded beyond my most optimistic expectations. I thank Dr. Wesley Nyborg and Dr. Marvin Ziskin for the enormous number of hours and intellectual effort that they contributed to this issue. I believe every physician involved with ultrasound scanning should have a copy of this book on his reference shelf.

Patients—especially those who are pregnant, and in light of the recent sensational news stories—have a right to question their physician about safety. These questions, however, may be difficult to answer without ready access to the information presented here. I believe that this book will become an invaluable source to physicians and sonographers, as well as to our patients.

Kenneth J.W. Taylor, M.D.

Preface

The question of the safety of ultrasound is an extremely important one. This book has been created to provide physicians, sonographers, and other health professionals with a summary of clinically relevant information on the biological effects of ultrasound. The material presented should make the reader better informed and give him a better understanding of the problems in assessing the risk of a clinical examination.

Besides its relevance to safety, the subject of ultrasonic bioeffects has an intrinsic interest. Ultrasound interacts with any medium through which it passes, whether the medium be biological tissue or nonliving matter. Some characteristics of the interactions are unique and fascinating. Cells, tissues, and cultures are altered, reversibly or irreversibly, in diverse ways. Some of the ultrasonically produced changes are expected (for example, as a result of heating), but most are not well understood. Studies of ultrasonic bioeffects offer surprises and intellectual challenge.

Under controlled conditions the bioeffects are beneficial. Ultrasonic therapy, hyperthermia, and surgery—all involving physiological change that is introduced for the patient's welfare—are assuming an increasing role in medicine. Physicians recommending or using these procedures need to be aware of their potential and their contraindications.

In diagnostic ultrasound, the average intensities are usually much less than those used in therapy. Nevertheless, the possibility that tissues may be affected, either for good or ill, cannot be ignored. Users will want to be aware of the current state of knowledge on biological effects, as well as the climate of opinion on the topic of safety.

In this volume there has been considerable communication between editors and contributors. We are grateful to the authors for their cooperation and for the quality of their contributions. The occasional differences of opinions expressed by different authors attest to their honesty and independence of thought. We have found the contributions stimulating and hope the readers will also. We also wish to thank Dr. Kenneth J.W. Taylor for his suggestions, and the editorial staff of Churchill Livingstone for their assistance.

Wesley L. Nyborg, Ph.D.
Marvin C. Ziskin, M.D., M.S. Bm.E.

1 Ultrasonic Bioeffects and Their Clinical Relevance: An Overview

MARVIN C. ZISKIN

I wrote this chapter at the suggestion of my co-editor to express my viewpoint, as a research physician, of the biological effects of ultrasound and their clinical relevance. The chapter was written after having read all of the other chapters in this book, and my comments have been guided by what each author has stated. The following is what I believe to be an overview of the salient points pertaining to each chapter.

The use of diagnostic ultrasound in medicine has been very popular for over 15 years. Literally millions of patients have had ultrasound examinations, and the number of such examinations increases each year. It is now estimated that over half of all pregnant women in the United States have at least one ultrasound examination during their pregnancies. This implies that soon over half of our entire population will have been exposed to ultrasound prior to birth.

Because of the vast exposure of the general population to ultrasound, any question of the possibility of adverse effects or harm becomes very important. This has certainly been a major concern of physicians from the very start and in spite of the fact that practicing physicians have identified no adverse effects arising from ultrasound examinations, clinical safety is and will always remain a concern. This is especially true for exposures to the fetus. Accordingly, considerable attention is given to the fetus in this book.

In order to appreciate and understand the literature on biological effects, it is necessary to know something of the underlying physics and the terminology used in ultrasound. Of especial importance is the ability to compare ultrasonic exposures intelligently. One needs to know that intensity is expressed in watts per square centimeter or milliwatts per square centimeter. And, because of the nonuniformity of an ultrasound beam, it is necessary to speak of spatial-average and spatial-peak intensities. When the ultrasound is pulsed, as is the case in virtually all diagnostic imaging, it is also necessary to distinguish between the temporal-peak intensity occurring during the "on" period and the temporal-average intensity which includes both the "on" and "off" periods in its computation. These latter two intensities may differ by a factor of 1,000 or more. Further explanation of the various intensities and other terminology is provided in Chapter 2 by Dr. Kremkau.

Without a knowledge of mechanisms, the myriad of ultrasonically induced biological effects is nothing more than a hodge-podge of disconnected empirical observations. In Chapter 3, Dr. Nyborg describes the mechanisms by which ultrasound interacts with biological tissues. These are divided into thermal and nonthermal mechanisms. The best-understood mechanism is thermal. At sufficiently high temporal-average intensities, ultrasound can cause significant temperature elevation in the tissues. Depending upon the circumstances, this temperature elevation may or may not be beneficial. With the exception of some Doppler systems, the average intensities of diagnostic instruments are very small and temperature elevations equaling one degree centigrade or greater are highly unlikely. Therefore, thermal effects arising out of these diagnostic applications do not appear to be of any consequence. However, the same cannot be said of cavitation. Cavitation is a nonthermal mechanism that occurs when gas bubbles are acted upon by a sufficiently intense ultrasound beam. In cavitation, energetic activity in the vicinity of the bubbles is greatly enhanced and is capable of disrupting cells and tissues. Whether or not cavitation occurs in diagnostic applications is not known. Theoretical considerations suggest that one should expect cavitation phenomenon resulting from the acoustic outputs of diagnostic instruments if appropriate-sized bubbles were present. Because of the bubbles generated in decompression illness, we know that preexisting microbubbles must exist in various places in the body. However, the exact sites and form of these microbubbles are not known. The potential danger from cavitation consists in the possibility that bubbles of an appropriate size would be in close vicinity to a sensitive structure in the body at a time when that structure was irradiated with an ultrasound beam. To date, we have no evidence that cavitation has ever occurred within the body during a diagnostic examination.

In vitro studies provide an important testing ground for hypotheses about ultrasonic interactions with living cells. An obvious appeal of these studies is the ability to isolate the factors under consideration. Single cells can be studied in isolation or permitted to grow as monolayers attached to a culture vessel surface, or to grow as free-floating multicellular aggregates or spheroids. Effects observed in these systems following exposure to ultrasound have included cell detachment, cell membrane structural alterations, aggregation, chromosomal changes, and cell death. However, the clinical relevance of these findings is uncertain. Perhaps the most meaningful statement made on this topic has been the American Institute of Ultrasound in Medicine (AIUM) statement on *In Vitro* Biological Effects which is presented below.

It is often difficult to evaluate reports of ultrasonically induced *in vitro* biological effects with respect to the clinical significance. The predominant physical and biological interactions and mechanisms involved in an *in vitro* effect may not pertain to the *in vivo* situation. Nevertheless, an *in vitro* effect must be regarded as a real biological effect. Results from *in vitro* experiments suggest new end-points and serve as a basis for design of *in vivo* experiments. *In vitro* studies provide the capability to control experimental variables and thus offer a means to explore and evaluate specific mechanisms. Although they may have limited applicability to *in vivo* biological effects, such studies can disclose fundamental intercellular or intracellular interactions. While it is valid for authors to place their results in context and to suggest further relevant investigations, reports which do more than that should be viewed with caution.

There is an important reason why it is so difficult to ascertain the clinical relevance of in vitro observations in ultrasound experiments. Nearly all of the effects observed has been associated with the presence of cavitation. Although cavitation is to be expected in in vitro preparations, it has not been known to occur in the diagnostic practice. The viscoelastic tissues of the body are significantly less conducive for the occurrence of cavitation. The in vitro ultrasound studies of single cells and multicellular spheroids are presented by Dr. Miller in Chapter 4.

The effects of ultrasound on blood and blood elements have been studied in both in vitro and in vivo preparations. These studies have concentrated on red blood cells, platelets, coagulation, functional effects of leukocytes, chromosomal investigations, and vascular effects, and are described by Dr. Williams in Chapter 5. The positive findings in these studies have occurred in in vitro preparations, or in in vivo preparations in which the applied intensities were significantly above diagnostic levels. An interesting potential health hazard exists when ultrasonic contrast agents containing microbubbles are injected into the bloodstream. It is conceivable that these bubbles, when within an ultrasonic beam of a diagnostic instrument, might provide a source for cavitational effects. In vitro studies have shown that cavitation of gas bubbles can induce platelet aggregation at diagnostic intensity levels. However, the available experimental evidence indicates that diagnostic and therapeutic intensities of ultrasound do not appear to damage platelets in vivo or initiate blood coagulation provided that excessive temperature elevations are avoided. Changes in phagocytic and bactericidal indexes of leukocytes have been shown to be affected by ultrasonic exposure in in vitro preparations. There was only one study that showed a positive in vivo effect. Following a 5-minute exposure at diagnostic ultrasound intensities to the spleen of mice, Anderson and Barrett showed alterations in the immune response to sheep erythrocytes. However, the changes noted were small compared to the capacity of the immune system to respond to potentially serious immunologic challenge, and two independent laboratories were not able to reproduce these findings.

Certainly, any adverse effects of ultrasound arising in clinical applications are of importance. Perhaps, those of greatest concern are the ones that would alter the genetic apparatus and induce changes that would be inherited from generation to future generation. Dr. Thacker, in Chapter 6, reviews the investigations in this area. In terms of clinical practice, the few definite reports of damage to the genetic material occurred at intensities that are well in excess of those used in diagnostic applications. On the basis of the currently available evidence, it seems very unlikely that current diagnostic applications will lead to any increase in the frequencies of inherited changes.

Laboratory animals provide an invaluable tool for observing the effects of ultrasound when applied to the intact organism. Early pioneering studies using intense ultrasound demonstrated the capability of ultrasound to produce destructive lesions in adult cat and rat brains. Other studies have shown ultrasound's capability for destroying tissue within various organs in a number of different laboratory animals. For example, ovarian and testicular tissue damage have been observed in mice following exposure to moderate intensity levels of ultrasound. Although such studies have greatly aided our understanding of what damage one might expect from intense and moderate ultrasonic exposure, additional studies at diagnostic intensity levels are required to ascertain better the potential risks of clinical examinations. The AIUM issued the following "Statement on Mammalian *In Vivo* Ultrasonic Biological Effects":

In the low megahertz frequency range there have been (as of this date) no independently confirmed significant biological effects in mammalian tissues exposed to intensities* below 100 mW/cm². Furthermore, for ultrasonic exposure times† less than 500 seconds and greater than 1 second, such effects have not been demonstrated even at higher intensities, when the product of intensity* and exposure time† is less than 50 J/cm².

In assessing risk, overly simplistic attitudes should be avoided. The 100 mW/cm² intensity mentioned in the AIUM's statement should not be treated as a magic number. Levels under this value do not guarantee "perfect" safety, and levels above this value may well be appropriate if they are needed to yield diagnostic information. In choosing procedures and equipment, the obligation is always present to balance benefit against risk. Investigations of ultrasound bioeffects using laboratory animals are presented in Chapter 7 by Dr. O'Brien.

The structure most vulnerable to the effects of ultrasound may well be the unborn fetus. This has certainly been our experience with other environmental hazards such as ionizing radiation, and there is evidence to suggest that this would not be the case for ultrasound. Studies on the effect of ultrasound on the mammalian fetus are presented in Chapter 8 by Drs. Carstensen and Gates. A survey of the literature regarding effects of ultrasound on the mammalian fetus fails to reveal any clear evidence that diagnostic ultrasound presents a potential hazard. Although prolonged intrauterine temperature elevations are known to cause serious fetal damage, enough is known about the heating mechanism of ultrasound to rule out any significant elevation of temperature

---

* Spatial peak, temporal average as measured in a free field in water.
† Total time; this includes off-time as well as on-time for a repeated pulse regime.

during most diagnostic procedures. Cavitation, however, cannot be ruled out. The intensity thresholds for the occurrence of transient cavitation using milli-second-length pulses are of the order of 10 W/cm². To be very conservative, one might suggest that only temporal-peak intensities below this threshold be used in diagnostic procedures. This, of course, would greatly reduce any potential hazard resulting from a cavitational mechanism. However, it remains to be seen if ultrasound instrumentation can provide diagnostically adequate images with such low peak intensities.

The clinical conditions under which the human fetus is exposed to ultrasound are presented by Dr. Hohler in Chapter 9. Diagnostic ultrasound has become a vital part of obstetric practice. No other imaging technique currently available can replace or rival the capabilities of diagnostic ultrasound for rapid provision of diagnostically efficacious information. According to a National Institute of Health Consensus Panel Report, there are 27 obstetric conditions in which diagnostic ultrasound is indicated. There are no known side effects or contrain-dications to the use of diagnostic ultrasound on the human pregnant woman or fetus. Nevertheless, it is considered prudent to minimize all exposures to that necessary to obtain the desired clinical information.

Chapter 10, written by Dr. Ziskin, presents the epidemiology of human exposure to ultrasound. No matter how many laboratory experiments show a lack of effect from diagnostic ultrasound, it will always be necessary to study directly its effect on human populations before any definitive statement regarding risk can be made. The collective experiences of physicians performing millions of patient examinations over the past 15 years and several large clinical surveys have not disclosed any clear example of an adverse effect. While this is most reassuring, it is not known how diligently these effects were being looked for. Although any gross acute adverse effect would appear to be most unlikely, subtle effects, such as minor chemical changes and minor behavioral changes, long-term delayed effects, and certain genetic effects could easily es-cape detection. Statistical considerations point out the difficulty in detecting adverse effects which are rare. Sample sizes required for statistical significance may become enormous if the effect is small. For example, a sample size of approximately ½ million individuals would be required to detect an increase in the frequency of occurrence of an abnormality from 10 to 10.1 percent. However, large clinical surveys even if negative, can provide an upper limit to the risk attendant to an ultrasound examination.

Not all biological effects are harmful. Ultrasound has been used for over 40 years as a therapeutic agent, mainly as a means of stimulating the repair of soft tissue injuries and relieving pain. The average intensities employed are typically many times higher than those used in most diagnostic applications. At these higher levels, significant heating of deep tissues is possible, particularly those with high acoustic absorption coefficients. This selective deep heating of tissues is the mechanism responsible for most of the beneficial therapeutic application of ultrasound described in Chapter 11 by Dr. Dyson. However, there is increasing evidence that nonthermal mechanisms may be involved in the production of several of the beneficial effects. Acceleration of wound healing and of bone repair are two effects for which the mechanisms are believed to be nonthermal. Although ultrasonic therapy has an excellent record of safety when correctly used, its very effectiveness in modifying tissue makes it a potentially dangerous modality if used inappropriately. Several contraindications and precautions associated with ultrasonic therapy should be observed. For example, terminate the treatment if the patient experiences pain, never treat anesthetic areas, and never irradiate the pregnant uterus with therapeutic levels of ultrasound.

Within the last 2–3 years, there has been a great resurgence of interest in the ability of local hyperthermia to destroy selectively cancer cells in vivo. Temperatures of 42.5°C or higher for 20–30 minutes appear to be necessary for tumoricidal effects; and several sessions, preferably 2 or more days apart, seem to be required for significant tumor regression. Ultrasonic and electromagnetic radiations are the two principal modalities used for this purpose. The use of ultrasound for cancer therapy is presented by Dr. Lele in Chapter 12.

The feasibility of using ultrasound for brain surgery was first demonstrated 40 years ago. By using focused transducers to produce very high ultrasonic intensities (10 W/cm² and higher), it is possible to destroy selectively deep structures while leaving intervening tissue undamaged. Furthermore, the tissue modification is accomplished without damage to blood vessels so there is no hemorrhage. Surgical applications of ultrasound, described by Dr. Wells in Chapter 13, have been applied to the treatment of Parkinson's disease, pituitary gland disease, vestibular surgery, and cataract surgery. Additional applications include calculus disintegration and dental scaling.

In the interest of caution and the public welfare, various professional groups and governmental agencies have adopted or proposed standards and guidelines for manufacturers and users of medical ultrasound equipment. Chapter 14, written by Drs. Ziskin and Nyborg, presents the activities of organizations in this area. Standards for equipment have been called for by various countries and organizations. In the United States, specifications on exposure parameters are provided for all ultrasonic therapy equipment as required by law. For diagnostic equipment the specifications are made public only when the manufacturer chooses to do so. In an effort to encourage publication of the data for diagnostic equipment, the AIUM awards certificates of commendation to manufacturers who make reliable information on exposure parameters conveniently available to the medical community. Advice has varied concerning the desirability of placing upper limits on output intensities of diagnostic equipment, with differing levels suggested for fetal Doppler equipment and pulse echo devices. Guidelines for medical practice have been issued by the National Council on Radiation Protection relative to both diagnostic and therapeutic application of ultrasound. A National Institute of Health Consensus Panel stated that the data on clinical efficacy and safety do not allow a recommendation for the routine screening of pregnant women at this time. The New Jersey State Department of Health recommended that the performance of amniocentesis ideally should be performed within an ultrasound facility. Many, if not all, organizations have recommended that ultrasound scans be limited to those with medical indications and not undertaken for social or frivolous reasons.

The personal viewpoints of selected ultrasound authorities are presented in the second half of Chapter 14. These viewpoints are important because physicians and other ultrasound users are probably influenced at least as much by personal opinions and advice from respected individual colleagues as by the deliberations of committees and agencies. The thoughtful comments of these authorities are well worth reading.

2 Physical Considerations

FREDERICK W. KREMKAU

Ultrasound is sound, with which we are familiar, but at a frequency (to be discussed later) that is higher than the human hearing range. Diagnostic ultrasound frequencies are in the 1–15 MHz range. Within this frequency range, imaging depth and resolution requirements are reasonably met. Ultrasound imaging is accomplished by producing short (approximately 1 μs) pulses of ultrasound which are reflected and scattered by tissues and tissue interfaces. The echoes which return to the sound source are detected and displayed in a cross-sectional anatomy format. Continuous sound is used for flow measurements and fetal monitoring during labor.

Biological-effects experiments utilize ultrasound sources of two types: (1) experimental laboratory systems which have flexibility in the parameters of the ultrasound produced and (2) diagnostic imaging or flow-detection equipment designed for clinical purposes.

In this chapter I will describe the devices that produce ultrasound, the ultrasound field patterns produced, the various parameters that are used to characterize continuous and pulsed ultrasound, the weakening of the sound as it travels, and reflection of ultrasound at media boundaries. More complete treatments of this material are available in textbook form.[1-6]

TRANSDUCERS AND BEAMS

A transducer is a device that converts energy from one form to another. Ultrasound transducers convert electrical energy to ultrasound and vice versa. They utilize the piezoelectric effect which is descriptive of certain materials which when deformed will develop a voltage across them or, conversely, expand or contract when a voltage is applied. Synthetic ceramics, most commonly formulations of lead zirconate titanate, and crystalline quartz, are commonly used for transducer materials. The transducer material is normally cut in the shape of a disc whose thickness determines the operating frequency and whose diameter determines characteristics of the ultrasound beam. These transducers are air-backed (have air behind the rear face of the transducer inside the transducer assembly) when designed for continuous ultrasound production. In order to produce short ultrasound pulses, transducers must have damping material inserted directly behind the rear face of the transducer. This allows short pulses to be produced but also decreases the efficiency of the transducer.

For continuous ultrasound production, an alternating voltage of the appropriate frequency is applied to the transducer resulting in the continuous production of ultrasound of the same frequency. To generate ultrasound pulses, short bursts (a few cycles of alternating voltage) are repeatedly applied to the transducer, producing the pulses. A second method of producing ultrasound pulses is to apply a very short (small fraction of a microsecond) electrical voltage impulse to the transducer. This results in a few cycles of ultrasound produced by the transducer. The more the damping, the shorter the ultrasound pulse produced in the latter case. This means of pulse production is referred to by the term *shock-excitation*. It is analogous to striking a bell with a hammer.

Ultrasound pulses contain frequencies other than the dominant or center frequency (which is usually equal to the operating frequency of the transducer). The range from the lowest to the highest frequency present in the pulses is called the *bandwidth*. The bandwidth divided by center frequency is called the *fractional bandwidth*. The reciprocal of fractional bandwidth is the *quality factor* or *Q*.

The ultrasound produced by the transducer travels away from the front face in the direction in which the transducer is pointing. The sound is collimated into a region called the beam as shown in Figure 2.1. This is commonly divided into two regions called the near field or near zone and the far field or far zone. The near zone is a region of spatially fluctuating ultrasound strength. The far zone has a much smoother distribution of ultrasound within it. The near zone extends out from the face of the transducer to a distance L:

$$L = D^2/4\lambda$$

where D is transducer diameter and λ is wavelength (described later). The beam diverges in the far zone with divergence angle ϕ (in degrees):

$$\phi = 70\lambda/D$$

for D larger than 10λ. Most of the acoustic energy which propagates outward from the transducer passes within the divergence angle (Fig. 2.1).

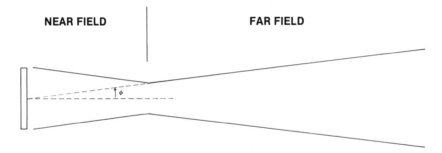

NEAR FIELD   **FAR FIELD**

FIG. 2.1   Ultrasound beam from an unfocused disc transducer.

Beam focusing is accomplished by curving the transducer surface or by attaching a lens to the transducer. Focusing is done in ultrasound imaging to improve lateral resolution in the focal region. It is used in biological effects experiments to increase the intensity produced (in the focal region) and/or to localize the high intensity to a particular anatomic site. The focal length of a focused transducer is the distance from the center of the transducer to the center of the focal region.

CONTINUOUS-WAVE ULTRASOUND

Sound is a temporal and spatial variation in acoustic variables (pressure, density, temperature, particle displacement, particle velocity, and particle acceleration). In a traveling wave the variations propagate through space at a speed characteristic of the medium. Continuous-wave (CW) sound (Fig. 2.2) is described by several parameters.

Frequency

The number of times that an acoustic variable goes through a complete variation (cycle) in 1 second is called the *frequency*. The unit of frequency is hertz which equals 1 cycle/s. Diagnostic ultrasound commonly operates in the range 1–15 MHz (megahertz or millions of hertz).

Period

The time required for a cycle to occur is called the *period*. Period and frequency are inversely related:

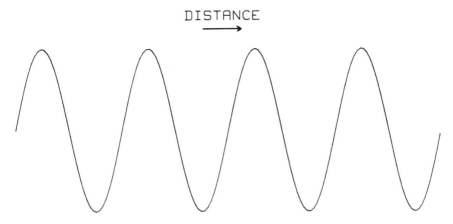

DISTANCE

FIG. 2.2 Continuous-wave sound is a series of cycles of varying pressure (or any other acoustic variable).

$$T = 1/f$$

where f is frequency and T is period.

Wavelength

The length of a cycle in space is called the *wavelength*. It decreases as frequency increases.

Propagation Speed

The speed with which ultrasound travels through a medium is called the *propagation speed*. It is determined by the density and stiffness or compressibility of the medium. Frequency, wavelength, and propagation speed are related to each other:

$$c = f\lambda$$

where λ is wavelength and c is propagation speed. Propagation speeds in soft tissues, cell suspensions, and liquid media are generally around 1,500 m/s or 1.5 mm/μs. Values in solids are higher while those in gases are lower.

Impedance

A second parameter that is determined by the medium is called the *impedance*. It is equal to density times propagation speed and is important when considering reflections at boundaries (discussed later). As with propagation speeds, impedance values are low, medium, and high for gases, liquids, and solids, respectively.

PULSED ULTRASOUND

The ultrasound used for medical imaging and applied in many biological-effects experiments is not CW but pulsed (Fig. 2.3). The description of pulsed ultrasound requires several parameters in addition to those discussed above.

Pulse Repetition Frequency

The *pulse repetition frequency* (*PRF*) is the number of pulses occurring per second. For typical scanning equipment the PRF is about 1,000 s^{-1}.

DISTANCE

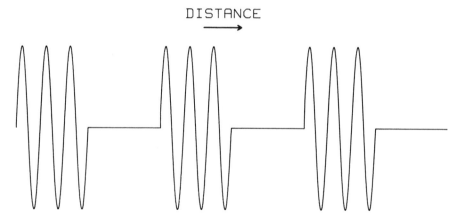

FIG. 2.3 *Pulsed ultrasound* is a series of pulses each containing one or more cycles of varying pressure (or any other acoustic variable).

Pulse Repetition Period

The *pulse repetition period* (*PRP*) is the time from the beginning of one pulse to the beginning of the next. Pulse repetition frequency and pulse repetition period are inversely related:

$$PRP = 1/PRF$$

Pulse Duration

Pulse duration is the length of time required for a pulse to occur. It is equal to the period times the number of cycles in the pulse:

$$PD = nT = n/f$$

where PD is pulse duration and n is the number of cycles in the pulse.

Duty Factor

The *duty factor* is the fraction of time that pulsed ultrasound is on. It is determined by the pulse duration and pulse repetition period:

$$DF = PD/PRP = PD \times PRF = nT \times PRF$$

where DF is duty factor.

AMPLITUDE AND INTENSITY

In previous sections we have considered the parameters that describe the temporal and spatial characteristics of CW and pulsed ultrasound. We have yet to introduce terms which relate to how large the variations are during a cycle. The maximum deviation from the normal value for an acoustic variable which occurs during a cycle is called the *amplitude*. The term "amplitude" may be applied to pressure, to displacement, to particle velocity, and to other acoustic variables, so that any given CW or pulsed ultrasound field may be described by several amplitudes. In each case, the appropriate unit is determined by the variable considered.

Energy-related quantities, especially power and intensity, are very important. These are discussed below as they apply to a beam of ultrasound in which energy travels outward from a source transducer into a homogeneous medium, such as water. Complications, such as those caused by reflections, are taken up later.

Power

The *acoustic power* of an ultrasound beam is the time rate of passage of energy through the beam cross-section. It is given in units of watts (W) or milliwatts (mW).

Intensity

Intensity is equal to the acoustic power passing through a cross-section divided by the area of the cross-section. It is also related to amplitude:

$$I = P/A = p^2/2z$$

where I is intensity, P is power, A is area, p is pressure amplitude, and z is impedance.

Because power and intensity are not uniformly distributed throughout the beam or in time (in the case of pulsed ultrasound), several intensities must be defined.

Spatial-Average Temporal-Average Intensity

The *spatial-average temporal-average* $(SATA)$ intensity is the value calculated when the total power in an ultrasound beam is divided by the beam area and averaged over the pulse repetition period (for pulsed ultrasound). When evaluated at the transducer face this is called I_t. The quantity I_t ranges from less than 1 up to about 20 mW/cm² for diagnostic scanning and fetal Doppler equipment, from 0.05 to 0.5 W/cm² for peripheral vascular Doppler equipment and from 0.5 to 3 W/cm² for therapy equipment.

Spatial-Peak Temporal-Average Intensity

The *spatial-peak temporal-average* (*SPTA*) intensity is the maximum value of intensity occurring in the beam averaged over the pulse repetition period (for pulsed ultrasound) in the beam. Typical values for diagnostic equipment are listed in Table A.1.

Spatial-Average Temporal-Peak Intensity

The *spatial-average temporal-peak* (*SATP*) intensity is the maximum value occurring in time of the spatially averaged intensity. For pulses of constant amplitude (Fig. 2.3) the SATP intensity is just the spatial average of the intensity during a pulse, and is equal to the SATA intensity divided by the duty factor.

Spatial-Average Pulse-Average Intensity

The *spatial-average pulse-average* (SAPA) intensity is the spatially averaged intensity averaged also over the pulse duration (for pulses of nonconstant amplitude). The distinction between temporal peak (TP) and pulse average (PA) values is necessary because very short pulses are normally not of constant amplitude (Fig. 2.4). Also, the longer pulses used in physical therapy are often not constant. For constant-amplitude pulses (Fig. 2.3) TP and PA intensities are the same.

DISTANCE

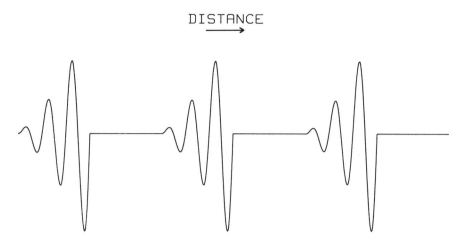

FIG. 2.4   Pulses produced by electrical shock excitation of a damped transducer contain cycles of differing amplitudes.

Spatial-Peak Pulse-Average Intensity

The *spatial-peak pulse-average* (*SPPA*) intensity is the maximum intensity in the beam averaged over the pulse duration (for pulses of nonconstant amplitude). Typical values for diagnostic equipment are listed in Table A.1.

Spatial-peak values may be two to four times greater than spatial-average values for unfocused transducers while for focused transducers they may be greater by a factor of 100.

Maximum Intensity

The *maximum intensity* (I_m) is the maximum value occurring in space (within the beam) and time. Typical values range from less than 1 up to 300 W/cm² for scanning equipment. For typical diagnostic pulses, I_m is greater than the SPPA intensity by a factor varying from 1.5 to 3.0.

ATTENUATION

As sound travels through a medium, its amplitude and intensity (ignoring the effects of focusing) decrease (Fig. 2.5). This weakening of the ultrasound is called *attenuation*. It is caused by scattering of sound in heterogeneous media, reflection of sound at interfaces, and conversion of sound energy to heat (absorption). Absorption is discussed in Chapter 3. Attenuation per unit distance of sound travel is called the attenuation coefficient. It is commonly expressed in decibels (dB) per centimeter. In soft tissues, the attenuation in dB/cm is approximately equal to half the frequency in megahertz. In liquids, attenuation is generally proportional to frequency squared. Table 2.1 describes decibel values, as they relate to intensity reduction. Table 2.2 describes attenuation values for tissues. Table 2.3 describes attenuation values for water.

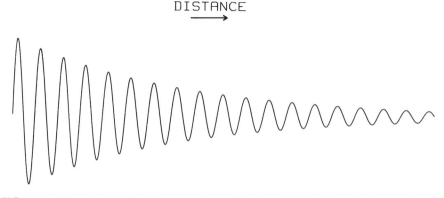

DISTANCE

FIG. 2.5 *Attenuation* is the decrease of amplitude and intensity of ultrasound as it travels through a medium.

TABLE 2.1 Intensity reduction in terms of decibels

Decibels (dB)	Intensity Reduction (%)
1	21
2	37
3	50
4	60
5	68
6	75
7	80
8	84
9	87
10	90
20	99

TABLE 2.2 Attenuation in tissue

Frequency (MHz)	Approximate Attenuation in Tissue (dB/cm)	Intensity Reduction in 1-cm Path (%)	Intensity Reduction in 10-cm Path (%)
1	0.5	11	68.4
2.25	1.0	21	90.0
3.5	2.0	37	99.0
5	2.5	44	99.7
7.5	4.0	60	99.99
10	5.0	68	99.999

TABLE 2.3 Attenuation in water

Frequency (MHz)	dB/cm
0.2	0.000088
0.5	0.00055
1.0	0.0022
2.0	0.0088
5.0	0.055
10.0	0.22

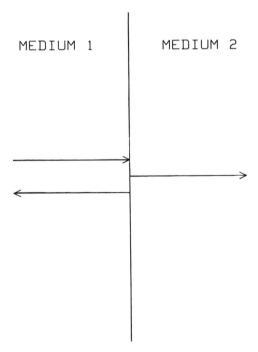

FIG. 2.6   Reflection of ultrasound at a boundary (perpendicular incidence).

REFLECTION

When ultrasound encounters a boundary between two media of differing impedances, a portion is reflected at the boundary. For the case where the incident sound direction is perpendicular to the boundary (Fig. 2.6), the intensity reflection coefficient (IRC, i.e., fraction of intensity reflected) depends upon the impedances as follows:

$$IRC = [(z_2 - z_1)/(z_2 + z_1)]^2$$

where IRC is the intensity reflection coefficient and z_1 and z_2 are media impedances. The fraction of intensity transmitted into the second medium is called the *intensity transmission coefficient (ITC)*:

$$ITC = 1 - IRC$$

For CW ultrasound or pulses of many cycles the incident and reflected sound from a boundary interfere to produce standing waves. In standing waves, positions of maximum and minimum pressure and particle velocity occur and remain

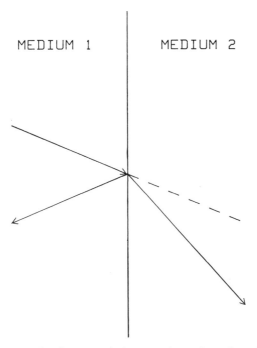

MEDIUM 1   MEDIUM 2

FIG. 2.7   Reflection and refraction of ultrasound at a boundary (*oblique incidence*).

fixed in space. The maxima are separated by a distance of ½ wavelength, and minima by the same distance.

In the case where the incident sound direction is not perpendicular to the boundary (Fig. 2.7), IRC and ITC depend on the angles involved as well as the impedances. Refraction, a change in the direction of the (unreflected) ultrasound as it crosses a boundary, is caused by differing propagation speeds on either side of the boundary.

EXPOSURE DATA

The American Institute of Ultrasound in Medicine (AIUM)[7] has developed a list of important ultrasound exposure parameters which have significant bearing on a reader's ability to evaluate a published biological-effects report. This list is given in Table 2.4.

The AIUM Manufacturers' Commendation Award (see Chapter 14 of this volume) requires the specification of several parameters[8] previously described in this chapter. They are listed in Table 2.5.

TABLE 2.4   AIUM recommended exposure parameter list for bioeffects reports

A. Ambient conditions
   1. Temperature
   2. Pressure
   3. Physiologic/biochemical state
   4. Mobility
   5. Specimen size

B. Exposure arrangements
   1. Ultrasonic beam configuration relative to specimen
   2. Coupling medium and arrangement
   3. Presence of gas
   4. Standing wave, reflection, refraction, diffraction

C. Transducer
   1. Geometrical configuration
   2. Beam configuration
   3. Moving or fixed beam
   4. Spatial beam shape
   5. Beam width (3 dB, 6 dB)

D. Ultrasound parameters
   1. Intensity (I_m, SPTA, SATP, SATA, SPPA)
   2. Total power
   3. Acoustic pressure
   4. Frequency
   5. Frequency bandwidth
   6. Shock parameter

E. Delivery data
   1. Pulse repetition frequency
   2. Pulse duration
   3. Duty factor
   4. Exposure time
   5. Repeated exposure parameters

F. Dosimetry and calibration
   1. Ultrasound parameters in free field or at site of interest
   2. Calibration technique (direct or indirect)
   3. Precision (repeatability)
   4. Accuracy (measured against standard true value)

G. Observation
   1. Temperature increase
   2. Cavitation
   3. Radiation-force effects
   4. Streaming

H. Instrumentation
   1. Manufacturer
   2. Model
   3. Modifications

TABLE 2.5   Parameter list for AIUM manufacturer's commendation award

1. Ultrasonic power
2. Spatial-peak temporal-average intensity
3. Spatial-peak pulse-average intensity (if pulsed)
4. Center frequency of transducer assembly
5. Fractional bandwidth of transducer assembly (if pulsed)
6. Pulse repetition frequency (if pulsed)
7. Focal length and focal area, if focusing transducer assembly
8. Entrance beam dimensions

REFERENCES

1. Kremkau FW: Diagnostic Ultrasound: Principles, Instrumentation, and Exercises, 2nd Ed. Grune & Stratton, Orlando, 1984

2. McDicken WN: Diagnostic Ultrasound: Principles and Use of Instruments, 2nd Ed. John Wiley and Sons, New York, 1981

3. Wells PNT: Biomedical Ultrasonics. Academic Press, New York, 1977

4. Wells PNT, Ziskin MC (eds): New Techniques and Instrumentation in Ultrasonography. Clinics in Diagnostic Ultrasound, Vol. 5. Churchill Livingstone, New York, 1980

5. Fry FJ (ed): Ultrasound: Its Applications in Medicine and Biology. Elsevier, New York, 1978

6. Edmonds PD (ed): Ultrasonics. Methods of Experimental Physics, Vol. 19. Academic Press, New York, 1981

7. American Institute of Ultrasound in Medicine Bioeffects Committee. J Ultrasound Med 2:R14, 1983

8. American Institute of Ultrasound in Medicine Commendation of Manufacturers. J Ultrasound Med 2:R6, 1983

3 Mechanisms

WESLEY L. NYBORG

In this volume many examples are given of changes in living systems brought about by exposure to ultrasound. Most of the reliable information on these changes has come from controlled laboratory experiments (Chapters 4–8), although some is from observations made by physicians in the course of clinical practice using ultrasonic therapy, hyperthermia, or surgery (Chapters 10–13). In some of the laboratory studies, the work has not been confined to observations of biological effects, but has also included attempts to seek out their causes. Determining the cause, or *mechanism,* is not only satisfying intellectually but has considerable practical value. With knowledge of the mechanisms for biological effects of ultrasound, the chances are improved for predicting and controlling the outcome of exposures.

THERMAL MECHANISM

Physical Considerations

As an intermediate cause of biological effects produced by ultrasound, *heat production* is one of the most important processes that occurs during ultrasonic exposure of animal tissue. As explained in Chapter 2, sound is attenuated as it travels through a medium; that is, its intensity decreases as it travels. Part of the attenuation is caused by conversion of sonic energy into heat, that is, by absorption; the remainder is from other causes, such as beam deflection and scattering. That part of an attenuation coefficient that results from heat production is called the absorption coefficient. For a homogeneous medium such as water (Table 2.3) all of the attenuation comes from absorption; the coefficients for absorption and attenuation are then equal. In a tissue (which, of course, is not homogeneous) some of the attenuation is a result of ultrasonic energy being redirected, so that it is lost from the ultrasound beam. This redirection is a consequence of reflection, refraction, and scattering at interfaces such as organ boundaries and walls of blood vessels. Hence for tissues the absorption coefficient is, in general, less than the attenuation coefficient. Although it has been shown recently for liver[1] (and may be true also for other soft tissues) that the difference is not very large at frequencies below 5 MHz, it probably becomes greater at higher frequencies.

Quantitative estimates of sonic heating at any location are easily made, by means of the following formula.

$$\text{Heating rate} = 0.055\,\alpha I \tag{1}$$

Here the terms are defined as:

Heating rate = local rate of heat production in calories per cubic centimeter
of exposed tissue per second (cal/cm^3 s)

α = absorption coefficient in decibels per centimeter (dB/cm); its
value depends on the frequency and on the tissue.

I = local time-averaged intensity in watts per square centimeter
(W/cm^2)

For example, we see from Table 2.2 that a typical value of the absorption coefficient for soft tissue at a frequency of 3.5 MHz is 2.0 dB/cm. If the local (time-averaged) intensity is 0.1 W/cm^2 we see from Equation (1) that the heating rate is (0.055 × 2.0 × 0.1) or 0.011 cal/cm^3 s. For tissues the heat capacity is approximately the same as for water (within about 10%); thus one calorie of heat added to 1 cm^3 of tissue raises its temperature by about 1°C. It follows for the example just given that the ultrasonically produced heat causes the local temperature to rise at a rate of 0.011°C/s or 0.7°C/min.

However, the numbers just cited give only the initial rate. As time goes on, the rate decreases; that is, while the temperature of the sonated tissue continues to rise, it does so less and less rapidly. This is because the sonically generated heat is transported to cooler regions. Part of the transport is accomplished by blood flow, that is, by *perfusion* (alternatively called *convection*), and the remainder is a result of heat *conduction* (alternatively called *diffusion*); the latter occurs even in a motionless medium.

In Figure 3.1 is a curve showing how the temperature rises at some point in a tissue exposed to ultrasound. The trends already described are exhibited. When the time is zero (at the left extreme of the graph) the ultrasound is applied and the temperature begins to rise. At first it rises at a nearly constant rate; the temperature during this initial period is approximately T_i and is greater than the initial temperature by an amount about equal to the heating rate given in Equation (1), multiplied by the time in seconds. As time goes on the curve flattens out, that is, the rate of temperature rise decreases. After a very long time the temperature approaches ever more closely, but never exceeds, a limiting value called the "final temperature" in Figure 3.1.

It is shown elsewhere, for example, in a report of the National Council on Radiation Protection and Measurements (NCRP),[2] that the final temperature rise and the "rise time" (the time required to reach an appreciable fraction, e.g., 50%, of the final temperature rise) are dependent on a number of factors. For an unfocused continuous beam, assumed for simplicity to be uniform,

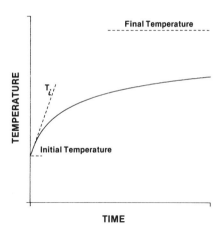

FIG. 3.1 Typical plot of temperature versus time at a point in a tissue exposed to ultrasound. The dotted straight line labeled T_i applies at first, and would apply indefinitely if there were no transport of heat by conduction or perfusion.

the final temperature rise increases (1) with increasing intensity, (2) with increasing absorption coefficient, and (3) with increasing beam diameter. Since the absorption coefficient increases with frequency and varies with tissue type, so does the final temperature rise.

The rise time increases with increasing beam diameter, but does not depend on the intensity or the absorption coefficient.

As an example,[2] consider a beam of intensity 0.2 W/cm², diameter 1.2 cm, and frequency 5 MHz propagating in a tissue similar to liver. The final temperature rise at a point 2 cm from the point of entry of the beam into tissue was calculated to be 3.0°C and the time required to reach half of this value was estimated to be about 300 seconds. In this calculation heat conductivity was taken into account, but not perfusion. In tissue well provided with blood flow as a coolant, the final temperature rise might be less by as much as a factor of 2 or more, and the rise time would be reduced.

Biological Effects of Heat

The animal body responds to temperature elevation in a variety of ways; some of these are familiar while others are less so. It is pointed out in Chapters 11, 12, and 13 of this volume that for many of the therapeutic and surgical applications of ultrasound the mechanism is thermal. This means that for these applications heat produced by nonacoustic means will cause the same response as does the ultrasound, provided that the thermal conditions are the same. To anticipate the possibilities for biological effects of ultrasound produced via a thermal mechanism it is useful to review briefly some known consequences of heating produced by other means.

Lehmann and De Lateur[3] list the following desirable effects of heat therapy in which the tissue temperature is maintained at a value from 40 to 45°C for a period of 5–30 minutes.

1. It increases the extensibility of collagen tissues.
2. It decreases joint stiffness.
3. It produces pain relief.
4. It relieves muscle spasms.
5. It assists in resolution of inflammatory infiltrates, edema, and exudates.
6. It increases blood flow.

In addition, hyperthermia is being used increasingly for the treatment of cancer. In some applications the entire body of a patient is maintained at a temperature of 41–42°C for several hours. In others, heat is supplied selectively to tumors, and higher temperatures are sometimes used.[3]

It is not well understood why the body responds as it does to temperature elevation, although there are a number of possible contributing factors. From physics and chemistry we know that the rates of fluid flow, of particle diffusion, and of biochemical reactions are all very temperature-dependent. Related to these facts are findings that raising the temperature affects passive membrane permeabilities, active transport processes, and metabolic rates. In addition, melting and other phase changes may result when the temperature is raised, with consequent changes in the functioning and integrity of cellular and subcellular structures.

Some of the therapeutic effects of heat are a consequence of vasodilation which, in turn, is brought about by various mechanisms. Among these is an interaction of blood vessels with histamine-like substances and bradykinin released by inflammatory reactions or by other means.[3]

For a typical biochemical reaction, catalyzed by an enzyme, its rate increases with increasing temperature until a peak value is reached, then declines as the enzyme becomes denatured. Thus, tissue metabolism may be speeded or slowed by heating, depending on the temperature.[3]

Applications of hyperthermia to cancer depend partly on the destructive capabilities of heat.[4] Elevated temperature causes tissue death at a rate that depends on the tissue and on the temperature. For example, when normal human skin tissue is maintained at a temperature of 45°C, thermal death occurs in about 2.5 hours. At lower temperatures the time required for thermal death is longer and at higher temperatures it is shorter. Specifically, a change of 1°C in temperature changes the time required by about a factor of 2.[5] This rough "factor-of-2-per-degree" rule applies rather generally to cells and tissues, although the time required for thermal death at a given temperature varies considerably with type and physiologic state of the cell or tissue.

Another mechanism for physiologic effects of hyperthermia is the inflammatory reaction, a response of the immune system, which follows tissue heating. While the response is stimulated by injury caused by the heat, the net effect may be beneficial.[6]

Caution has been advised in applying heat therapy to pregnant patients since temperature elevation is known to be a teratogenic factor.[3] Detailed findings on congenital defects produced by hyperthermia in guinea pigs have been reported by Edwards.[7, 8] In his experiments pregnant guinea pigs received "standard" 1-hour exposures to elevated temperature in an incubator set at 43.0–43.5°C. For a representative group of animals, internal ("core") temperatures were measured at intervals during the exposure and during recovery after removal from the incubator; results on the variation of temperature with time for a standard exposure are shown in Figure 3.2. It was estimated that in an exposure the core temperature was above normal (39.4°C) for about 90 minutes, above 41°C for at least 40 minutes, and above 42°C for at least 20 minutes. The temperature of the fetus was believed to be about the same as the core temperature, or slightly less.

Each pregnant guinea pig in the experiment received a set of standard exposures, one each day for 2, 4, or 8 successive days. These were administered at different stages of gestation, the entire gestational period being 68 days. Abortions (infrequent for controls) often occurred for females subjected to hyperthermia. For guinea pigs receiving a set of two exposures, abortions were most frequent when the exposures were on days 18 and 19 and then occurred for 6 of 11 exposed females; no abortions occurred for the 12 control animals which received no thermal exposure.

Fetal resorption also occurred, and was most frequent when exposures occurred during the period 11–15 days.

Abnormalities among newborn guinea pigs were observed as a result of exposures at a wide range of gestational age, but were most frequent when the exposures occurred at days 18–25. The most common defect was micrencephaly (reduced brain size), but hypoplastic (incompletely developed) digits, exomphalos (umbilical hernia), talipes (clubfoot), and others were also observed.

Detailed studies were made of reduced brain weight in progeny of guinea pigs exposed to hyperthermia. Included were experiments in which single 1-hour exposures were applied on day 21 of gestation. In these experiments different animals were subjected to different temperature-versus-time regimes by adjusting the incubator temperature to a range of selected values, from

FIG. 3.2   Core temperature in guinea pig during heat treatment (0–60 minutes) and after treatment (60–150 minutes). Points show mean observed temperature. Vertical lines through the points extend 1 standard deviation above and below the mean. (Redrawn from Edwards MJ: Congenital defects in guinea pigs: fetal resorptions, abortions and malformations following induced hyperthermia during early gestation. Teratology 2:313, 1969.)

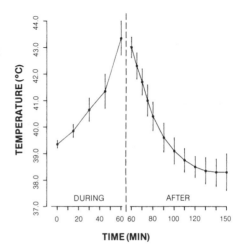

38 to 43°C. The time course of temperature was as shown in Figure 3.2, except that the maximum core temperature (which occurs at 60 minutes) was varied. Prenatal brain growth was found to be retarded when the maximum core temperature exceeded 41.8°C, about 2.5°C above normal. For each 1°C increase in maximum maternal core temperature the brain weight for a given total birth weight decreased by 0.23 g or about 8.4 percent.[8]

Experiments with other animals also show teratologic effects of heat. In a review of the subject Lele[9] points out that the dividing and differentiating cell populations of the embryo are susceptible to damage by heat (as well as other agents), especially at the stage of organogenesis. Lele cites results for a number of animals showing that systemic hyperthermia of 2.5–5°C above the normal temperature for the species, maintained for 1 hour or longer, causes abortion or fetal abnormalities.

Also for human beings there is evidence that hyperthermia is a teratogenic agent; this has been obtained by examining records of patients who experienced febrile illness during pregnancy. Smith et al.[10] examined eight patients in which maternal fever of 38.9°C (1.5°C above normal) or higher occurred during pregnancy, at 4–6 weeks gestation. He found for these patients patterns of malformations and brain dysfunction similar to each other as well as to patterns described by Edwards and others for the guinea pig and other animals. Furthermore, the results for these patients were similar even though the (infectious) cause of the fever varied with the individual.

Biological Effects of Ultrasound Mediated by Heat

The changes described above, which occur in a living system when its temperature is elevated by nonacoustic means, should also occur when the same temperature rise is produced by ultrasound. Examples of desirable changes are given in Chapters 11 to 13. There it is pointed out that ultrasonic techniques offer advantages over other methods of applying heat to a patient. With ultrasound the heat is generated within the tissue rather than at its surface. Also the spatial distribution of heat can be controlled by manipulation of focused beams.

As might be expected, undesirable effects of temperature elevation can also occur, whether the heat is generated by ultrasound or by other means. Possibilities relative to effects of ultrasound on the fetus in animal experiments are discussed in Chapters 7 and 8. Development abnormalities would be expected if, in applying ultrasound to a pregnancy, the temperature of the fetus were to be elevated by several degrees and maintained at that level for an extended period. However, significant heating of the fetus is very unlikely in any usual application of ultrasound in diagnosis or therapy. Considerable insight on the possibilities here has come from laboratory experiments on mice[9, 11] and guinea pigs.[12] In these it was found that ultrasound can indeed elevate the fetal temperature enough to affect the fetus significantly. However, the conditions required to do so are very different from those which exist when ultrasound is applied to a human patient. In the laboratory experiment the (continuous wave) intensity required was over 100 mW/cm^2 and was applied uniformly over the fetal body for a period of time extending from 10 to 90 minutes. The medical situation in diagnosis differs in that (1) the time-averaged intensity at the fetus is usually much less (usually by, at least, a factor of 4, and often by a much larger factor); (2) except during the first weeks of pregnancy, only a small part of the fetus is exposed to ultrasound at any given time; (3) the duration of exposure at any location is usually small; and (4) cooling mechanisms may be more effective in the medical application than they are in the laboratory situation.[2, 9] Nevertheless, users of medical ultrasound have been advised to err on the side of caution, and to avoid applying ultrasound to a pregnant woman in any way that might raise the fetal temperature significantly.[2]

NONTHERMAL MECHANISMS

While as shown above, heat can be an important intermediary when ultrasound affects a living system, there are numerous situations where heat plays only a minor role, or is not involved at all. These situations are known from experiments in which the time-averaged ultrasonic intensity is small, or the system is cooled, so that little or no temperature rise occurs.

Radiation Pressure

In a beam of ultrasound, such as is described in Chapter 2, oscillatory movements occur and the pressure varies in time and space. In addition to variations of the pressure above and below its mean value, which occur during each cycle, there are increments or decrements of its mean value. An increase of the mean pressure at a point in a sound field is called here the *radiation pressure* at that point. (Note: Usage of this term varies somewhat in the literature.) The value of the radiation pressure depends on the nature of the sound field and on its intensity. In nonuniform sound fields the radiation pressure varies from point to point. In an attenuated plane traveling wave (Fig. 2.5) the radiation pressure increases as the intensity decreases, that is, it increases with distance from the source. In a plane standing wave, the radiation pressure is greatest at pressure maxima and least at velocity maxima.[13] Gavrilov[14] as well as Foster and Wiederhold[15], have given evidence that pulses of radiation pressure produced in brain by pulses of ultrasound give rise to disturbances that can be sensed by the ear.

Radiation Force

Any body, large or small, suspended in a liquid and exposed to ultrasound is acted on by a net radiation force. In a plane traveling wave the force is in the direction of wave propagation and is proportional to the intensity. This fact forms the basis of important methods for measuring ultrasonic intensity and power.

In a standing wave the direction of the force on an object depends on its properties. Most biological cells move to the pressure minimum nearest them in a standing wave. Because of this a standing wave established in a cell suspension causes the cells to become concentrated in a series of planes one half wavelength apart. This appears to be the basis for a striking phenomenon discovered by Dyson et al.,[16] using an arrangement which permitted blood vessels of chick embryos to be observed visually while ultrasound was applied. Under ultrasound a series of equally spaced clear areas appeared as the red cells aggregated into bands separated by a distance of one-half wavelength. The banding itself was found to be usually reversible, but was sometimes accompanied by irreversible damage to the epithelium. The intensity required to produce the banding was in the vicinity of 1 W/cm² (spatial average in a continuous wave), a level typical of ultrasonic therapy. In medical practice the banding can be avoided by moving the transducer about during an application.

Acoustic Torque and Acoustic Streaming

When a nonuniform ultrasonic field is set up in a tissue, or cell suspension, or other medium, a steady twisting action called *acoustic torque* may be exerted on any small part of the medium. Cells or intracellular structures may be set into spinning motion, with significant biological consequences.[2]

In a liquid, acoustic torque acting on elements of the liquid itself induces a steady eddying motion called *acoustic streaming.* This motion is especially significant biologically in situations where cells or intracellular organelles in aqueous environments are subjected to eddying of very small scale called *acoustic microstreaming.*[2] The cells or organelles are affected by hydrodynamic stresses exerted by the microstreaming via the high velocity-gradients associated with it; examples and possibilities are discussed in Chapters 4, 5, and 11. Effects of microstreaming are to be expected primarily when small gas bubbles of appropriate size are present (discussed in the section Cavitation and Gas-Bubble Activity, below) or when special arrangements are used to simulate the action of gas bubbles.

Cavitation and Gas-Bubble Activity

When a suspension of cells or macromolecules is exposed to ultrasound without significant temperature change, any effects produced are likely to be mediated by undissolved gas. To be effective at sound frequencies in the megahertz range the gas must be in the form of small bubbles, pockets, or other bodies, with dimensions of the order of microns or smaller, stabilized against diffusion in pores, channels, cracks, and so forth. In an ultrasound field of sufficient pressure amplitude, these gaseous bodies may exert mechanical stresses on surrounding cells or other structures, or may generate chemical activity. There are many aspects to the behavior of small gaseous bodies in an ultrasound field, all of which can be included under the terms *cavitation* or *gas body activity.* [2, 17] Many examples of changes in biological cells or other systems caused by some form of cavitation are taken up in Chapters 4 and 5, and possibilities for cavitation effects are discussed further in Chapters 6, 8, 11, and 13. A distinction has been made between *stable* cavitation and *transient* cavitation: the former is an activity associated with volume oscillations of a gas bubble which, in a continuous sound field, continue for many cycles; the latter is a more violent activity associated with collapse of the bubble during a single cycle, or after a very small number of cycles.

Considerable insight on the significance of small gas bodies in an ultrasound field has come from experiments carried out in tissues of plants and insects, where small gas-filled channels are known to exist. In these experiments it is found that these tissues are indeed particularly vulnerable to ultrasound, *specifically because of the gaseous channels.* It is also found for the tissues with gas-filled channels that for a given time-averaged intensity a pulsed mode of ultrasound is much more damaging than a continuous mode. [2, 18, 19]

In other experiments, described in Chapter 5, membranes with small gas-filled pores are used to promote activity in ultrasonic exposure of cell suspensions. In these it was shown that cellular change can occur at very low ultrasonic intensity levels, less than 10 mW/cm^2, spatial peak, in a continuous-wave mode.

It is now well established that diagnostic ultrasound, as generated by widely used commercial equipment, will produce significant biological effects in selected situations where small gas bodies of appropriate size are present.

By contrast, there is no direct evidence at present that significant numbers of such critical gas bodies exist in living mammals. Neither is there present evidence that diagnostic ultrasound produces cavitation activity in mammals. (See also Chapter 8.)

SYNERGISM

In the above discussion we have treated thermal and nonthermal mechanisms separately. They may, however, act synergistically. For example, Krizan and Williams[20] have shown that red cells are lysed by mechanical shear at increasingly smaller stress values as the temperature increases. Thus ultrasonically produced hyperthermia and ultrasonically produced mechanical stresses may lead to biological changes which would not occur as a result of either mechanism alone.

CONCLUSION

The ability to anticipate conditions under which ultrasound will produce change in a living system is improved by understanding mechanisms which may be involved. Medically beneficial changes can be produced by ultrasonically produced heat if the acoustic conditions are suitably chosen; see Chapters 11–13. Harm can result from ultrasonic heating if conditions are inappropriate. As an example of the latter possibility: if intensities characteristic of therapeutic ultrasound were applied to the fetus for an extended period of time, harmful temperature elevation would be expected. However, deleterious heating effects would be very unlikely during an application of diagnostic ultrasound to the fetus; most commercial equipment intended for examining pregnancies is incapable of raising the fetal temperature significantly, no matter how long the ultrasound is applied. Users can assure themselves on this matter for their own equipment by examining applicable intensity data, such as those tabulated in Appendix A.

Nonthermal mechanisms by which ultrasound affects biological cells and organisms include mechanical stresses, such as are expressed via radiation forces and acoustic microstreaming. In specialized nonmammalian systems, when microscopic gas-filled channels or pores are present, ultrasound can cause significant effects via mechanical stresses, even at the low time-averaged intensity levels characteristic of diagnostic ultrasound. However, there is no accepted evidence that typical diagnostic ultrasound can produce similar effects in mammals.

REFERENCES

1. Parker KJ: Ultrasonic attenuation and absorption in liver tissue. Ultrasound Med Biol 9:363, 1983

2. National Council on Radiation Protection and Measurements Report No. 74, Biological Effects of Ultrasound: Mechanisms and Clinical Implications. National Council on Radiation Protection and Measurements, Washington, DC, 1983

3. Lehmann JF, DeLateur BJ: Therapeutic heat. p. 404. In Lehmann JF (ed): Therapeutic Heat and Cold. 3rd Ed. Williams and Wilkins, Baltimore, 1982

4. Storm FK (ed): Hyperthermia in Cancer Therapy. GK Hall Medical Publishers, Boston, 1983

5. Dickson JA, Calderwood SK: Thermosensitivity of new plastic tissues in vivo. p. 63. In Storm FK (ed): Hyperthermia in Cancer Therapy. GK Hall Medical Publishers, Boston, 1983

6. Dickson JA, Shah SA: Immunological aspects of hyperthermia. p. 487. In Storm FK (ed): Hyperthermia in Cancer Therapy. GK Hall Medical Publishers, Boston, 1983

7. Edwards MJ: Congenital defects in guinea pigs: fetal resorptions, abortions and malformations following induced hyperthermia during early gestation. Teratology 2:313, 1969

8. Edwards MJ: Congenital defects in guinea pigs: prenatal retardation of brain growth of guinea pigs following hyperthermia during gestation. Teratology 2:329, 1969

9. Lele PP: Revue: safety and potential hazards in the current applications of ultrasound in obstetrics and gynecology. Ultrasound Med Biol 5:307, 1979

10. Smith DW, Clarren SK, Harvey MAS: Hyperthermia as a possible teratogenic agent. J Pediatr 92:878, 1978

11. Stolzenberg SJ, Torbit CA, Edmonds PD, Taenzer JC: Effects of ultrasound on the mouse exposed at different stages of gestation: acute studies. Radiat Environ Biophys 17:245, 1980

12. Ziskin MC, Barnett SB, Edwards MJ: Fetal brain weight reduction following ultrasonic exposure in guinea pigs. J Acoust Soc Am 63 (S1):S28A, 1978

13. Nyborg WL: Physical principles of ultrasound. p. 1. In Fry FJ (ed): Ultrasound: Its Applications in Medicine and Biology. Part I. Elsevier, New York, 1978

14. Gavrilov LR, Tsirul'nikov EM, Shchekanov EE: Stimulation of auditory receptors by focused ultrasound. Sov Phys Acoust 21:437, 1976

15. Foster KR, Wiederhold ML: Auditory responses in cats produced by pulsed ultrasound. J Acoust Soc Am 63:1199, 1978

16. Dyson M, Pond JB, Woodward B, Broadbent J: The production of blood cell stasis and endothelial damage in the blood vessels of chick embryos treated with ultrasound in a stationary wave field. Ultrasound Med Biol 1:133, 1974

17. Coakley WT, Nyborg WL: Cavitation; dynamics of gas bubbles; applications. p. 77. In Fry FJ (ed): Ultrasound: Its Applications in Medicine and Biology. Part I. Elsevier, New York, 1978

18. Carstensen EL: Biological effects of low temporal-average-intensity, pulsed ultrasound. Bioelectromagnetics 3:147, 1982

19. Miller DL: The botanical effects of ultrasound: a review. Environ Exp Botany 23:1, 1983

20. Krizan JE, Williams AR: Biological membrane rupture and a phase transition model. Nature New Biol 246, 1973

4 In Vitro Studies: Single Cells and Multicell Spheroids

MORTON W. MILLER

IN VITRO SYSTEMS: PRO AND CON

The ready availability of a variety of in vitro cell systems and the ease with which they can be cultured and analyzed for a variety of end-points has led to a large number of reports in the area of ultrasound bioeffects. First, in vitro systems can involve cells that can be grown as monolayers attached to a culture vessel surface, as cells that remain suspended in the culture medium and do not attach to the vessel surface, and as cells that form multicellular aggregates, or "spheroids," and must be continuously stirred to keep them suspended in the culture medium. Second, all these cell systems can be grown under a variety of carefully controlled environmental conditions and thus avail themselves readily to investigations involving mechanisms of action of ultrasound involved in the production of biological effects. For example, controllable parameters include the medium's gas content, the age, number and size of cells, their position in the cell cycle, and their position in the sound field. Third, the variety of end-points which can be investigated is extensive and ranges from growth (simple increase in cell number with time) to cytogenetics [sister chromatid exchanges (SCE)] to DNA analyses (thymine base damage). Because of the presumed general absence of genetic differences between cells (they are usually all derived—"cloned"—from a single cell), variability between experiments can be minimal. Thus, the general outlook for in vitro studies is outwardly simplistic, with an apparent high degree of precision available to the investigator in terms of biological and physical variables.

The outward simplicity of these in vitro systems must, however, be weighed against the relevance of results obtained with these systems to in vivo cells and tissues and the potentially very complicated exposure apparatuses which produce fields not necessarily similar to those obtained with in vivo tissue insonation. For example, the ultrasound field inside an insonated test tube can be a complex combination of standing and traveling waves whereas with in vivo exposures there may be only traveling waves. It should be obvious that before results from in vitro experiments can be extrapolated to in vivo situations one must know at least the rudiments of the physical mechanism of action producing the in vitro effect.

EXPOSURE CONDITIONS

A problem with in vitro systems is that the investigator must generally use conditions which maintain the sterility of the system. Typically, then, the investigator must expose the cells in some sort of sterile container which allows for exposure of the cells to the ultrasound but which retains the aseptic conditions of the culture. The large variety of exposure conditions used in ultrasound treatment of in vitro cell systems is shown in Figures 4.1 and 4.2. Cells have been exposed while directly on the transducer [Fig. 4.2(1)], in culture medium contained in a test tube which was stationary [Fig. 4.1(1)], or rotated [Fig. 4.1(2)] with the transducer outside the tube [Fig. 4.1(1,2)], or faced down into the tube [Fig. 4.1(3)], in medium contained in a thin glass bubble [Fig. 4.1(4)], down into or up through a petri dish [Fig. 4.1(7,8)], in medium contained in a chamber with anechoic windows [Fig. 4.1(5)], through a rectangular culture vessel [Fig. 4.1(6)], by acoustic "activation" of bubbles within a gas-rich hydrophobic Nuclepore filter immersed in cell suspension [Fig. 4.2(4)], by vibrating wires [Fig. 4.2(5)], through anechoic Teflon "baggies" [Fig. 4.1(9)], directly on a coverslip [Fig. 4.2(2)], or under conditions which simply weren't specified [Fig. 4.2(6)]. Each of these conditions can significantly influence the incident sound field and thus potentially influence the experimental results.

The type of exposure vessel has a great influence on whether or not cells will be affected by the incident sound field. Sacks et al.,[1] for example, have shown that with an anechoic chamber, cells were not lysed with continuous-wave (CW) ultrasound of 1.1 MHz frequency and spatial-peak, temporal-average (SPTA) intensities (Chapter 2) up to 20 W/cm². Neither were they lysed with similar exposures in a polystyrene test tube [Fig. 4.1(1)] when it was kept stationary during insonation. When the tube was rotated [Fig. 4.1(2)], however, a dramatic increase in cell lysis occurred at the same or smaller SPTA intensities. Clarke and Hill[2] had shown in 1969 that tube rotation was necessary in order to achieve cell lysis at the lowest intensities, and others have since confirmed this effect. Church et al.[3] have provided a mechanistic insight into how this "rotation" effect occurs. When a polystyrene test tube is placed in a 1-MHz sound field, the field is perturbed by the tube. When the tube contains a dilute charcoal suspension, the particles collect in a series of planes one-half-wavelength apart (Fig. 4.3). This demonstrates that the tube exposure system produces a standing-wave field. In a nonrotating tube [Fig. 4.1(1)] containing in vitro biological cells and gas bubbles, the cells and lytically effective bubbles are segregated by the presence of a stationary wave pattern in the tube, the cells collecting at the pressure nodes, the effective bubbles at the pressure antinodes (Fig. 4.4). Without tube rotation bubbles caused little cell damage since no cells were near the bubbles. With tube rotation [Fig. 4.1(2)], however, the cells, being held by only a weak force, are swirled with the fluid past arrays of bubbles still trapped at the pressure maxima. The rotation

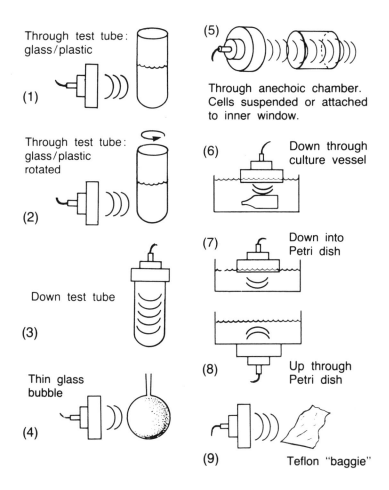

FIG. 4.1 Chamber systems for ultrasound exposure of in vitro cells.

brings the cells and effective bubbles into close proximity and lysis occurs. The general result for this system is that stabilized bubbles are demonstrated to be an important ingredient in the ultrasonically induced lysis of cells.

CAVITATION MECHANISM

That some form of cavitation mechanism is involved in most if not all of the reported in vitro effects is evident from a number of additional approaches. Ciaravino et al.[4] exposed Chinese hamster V-79 cells in rotating polystyrene tubes to 1-MHz CW ultrasound. In 5-minute exposures at spatial-peak intensities of 5 W/cm^2 and 10 W/cm^2, the percentage of intact cells was reduced to about 60 percent and 30 percent, respectively. These effects were eliminated

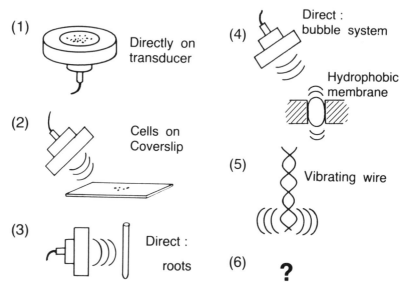

FIG. 4.2 Direct systems for ultrasound exposure of in vitro cells.

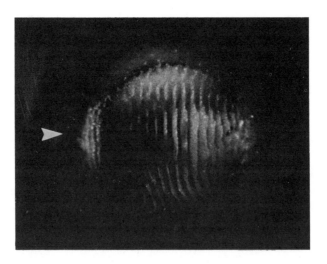

FIG. 4.3 A photograph from above of an aqueous suspension of an anion exchange resin in a continuous-wave insonated polystyrene test tube [Fig. 4.1(1)]. A light was beamed across the tube to highlight the "peaks" and shadow the "valleys" of the resin suspended by the standing-wave field in the exposure tube. The arrow indicates the direction of propagation of the sound field. (Reprinted with permission from Church CC et al: The exposure vessel as a factor in ultrasonically-induced mammalian cell lysis—II. Ultrasound Med Biol 8:299. Copyright 1982, Pergamon Press, Ltd.)

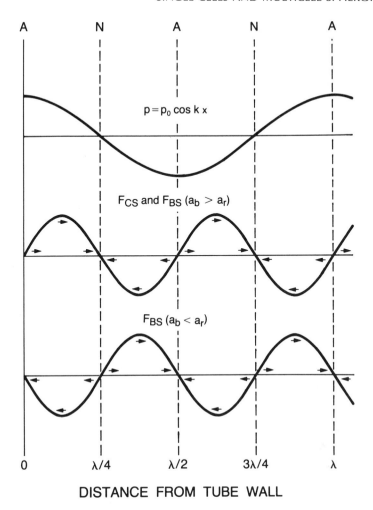

FIG. 4.4 The spatial relationships between the stationary wave acoustic pressure, p, and the forces on cells, F_{CS}, and bubbles, F_{BS}, due to the stationary wave. Amplitudes are arbitrary; arrows give the direction of the force at any position. Abbreviations: A = pressure antinode; a_b = bubble radius; a_r = bubble resonance radius; N = pressure node. (Reprinted with permission from Church CC et al: The exposure vessel as a factor in ultrasonically-induced mammalian cell lysis—II. Ultrasound Med Biol 8:299. Copyright 1982, Pergamon Press, Ltd.)

by increasing the ambient pressures to 1.5 atm and 2.0 atm, respectively. These data are consistent with transient cavitation as the mechanism for lysis and also with the rotating tube model described above.

In order for a bubble to undergo transient collapse it must expand to a maximum radius, which depends on the ratio of the acoustic pressure amplitude, P_a, to the ambient pressure, P_o.[5] In a plane traveling wave, intensity is related to pressure by the formula:

$$I = P_a^2/2\rho c$$

where ρ is the liquid density and c is the speed of sound (see Chapter 2). For intensities of 5 W/cm^2 and 10 W/cm^2 in water the values for P_a are 3.8 atm and 5.4 atm, respectively. The ratios are then

$$\frac{P_a}{P_o} = \frac{3.8}{1.5} = 2.5 \text{ (for I = 5 W/cm}^2)$$

$$\frac{P_a}{P_o} = \frac{5.4}{2.0} = 2.7 \text{ (for I = 10 W/cm}^2)$$

Thus, for two exposure intensities and ambient pressures needed to suppress cell lysis, there is approximate equality (average of 2.6) for this ratio. This result reinforces the notion that acoustic cavitation (in this example, specifically, transient cavitation) is responsible for cell lysis.

Several other kinds of evidence implicate cavitation in the induction of cell lysis. Cavitation can be detected by monitoring acoustic emission, particularly the first subharmonic frequency, from an insonated sample. Morton et al.[6] showed that a strong correlation was observed between cell damage and emitted subharmonic intensities; in the absence of a strong subharmonic signal no lysis was evident, and in the presence of subharmonic signals cell lysis occurred. Temperature dependence was shown by Armour and Corry[7] who exposed Chinese hamster ovary cells in an anechoic chamber to 1-MHz CW ultrasound at an intensity of 1 W/cm^2 (probably I_t, as defined in Chapter 2) and noted no effects on cell suspensions at 37°C, while at 3°C cell survival was greatly reduced at intensities between 1 and 3 W/cm.[2] That there was more gas dissolved in the medium equilibrated at 3°C than at 37°C suggests that the greater gas content promoted acoustic cavitation. Frequency dependence was shown by Chater and Williams[8] who exposed blood cells to CW ultrasound and noted an immediate effect on platelet shape at 1.5-MHz exposures of 1 W/cm^2 (I_t) but no effect for the same intensity at 3 MHz. Acoustic cavitation is known to be frequency-dependent, with a higher propensity at lower frequencies.

PARAMETERS FOR DETECTING "BIOLOGICAL EFFECTS"

There are, as might be surmised for in vitro experiments, a variety of parameters used to detect whether or not there has been a "biological effect." These parameters include cell lysis, cell viability, cell survival and growth, macromolecular (DNA, RNA, protein) syntheses, genetic and cytogenetic indexes, and membrane functions. Each of these parameters measures some aspect of living function. For example, cell lysis is determined by counting the number of cells before and after insonation. A cell that is physically destroyed, that is, whose membrane is ruptured, is said to be *lysed*. With cell lysis there are fewer intact cells after treatment than before. *Viability* is a measure of whether or not a cell is metabolically "alive." Just because a cell is apparently physically intact does not mean that it is viable. In general, parameters such as membrane function, macromolecular synthesis, and genetic and cytogenetic analyses measure different aspects of viability and can be used to indicate what are likely "targets" for ultrasound exposures. Cell lysis is a well-known phenomenon from use of sonic disintegrators, which operate at relatively low frequencies and high amplitudes and cause very evident acoustic cavitation. Cell lysis has also been reported to occur after insonation at clinically relevant frequencies (e.g., see Fu et al.,[9] Watmough et al.,[10] Kaufman et al.,[11] Coakley et al.,[12] and Moore and Coakley).[13] In all instances, as indicated above, results in this area strongly suggest acoustic cavitation as a mechanism involved in the ultrasonically induced lysis of cells.

Cell survival and growth have likewise been affected by insonation at clinically relevant frequencies.[11, 14, 15] In most instances the effects can be correlated with acoustic cavitation. The research of Chapman et al.,[15] however, contains results which do not appear completely compatible with an acoustic cavitation mechanism interpretation. True, cell survival and viability were altered more by a lower (0.75-MHz) than a higher (3-MHz) ultrasound frequency at a comparable intensity—this is consistent with a cavitational process. However, intracellular potassium content decreased more at the 3-MHz than at the 1.5-MHz exposure for the same intensity, and this effect was comparable for gassed and degassed insonated medium—these results do not appear compatible with a cavitation process and suggest the involvement of other mechanisms.

There are, unfortunately, a number of reports which do not allow for elucidation or deduction of a mechanism(s) of action of ultrasound on cells. The experiments in this category involve very complicated interactions of the sound field with the exposure chambers. For example, cells have been insonated on the bottom of a petri dish with the transducer coupled to the outer dish bottom, or without specification of the location of the transducer, or with the transducer irradiating down into a Petri dish. In the first and third situations, near-field inhomogeneities and reflections from air interfaces would greatly complicate the incident sound field.

WHERE ARE THE BIOLOGICALLY EFFECTIVE BUBBLES?

The question naturally arises as to where biologically effective bubbles are located. Are they in the medium surrounding the cells, or are the effects of bubbles rendered from within the cell. Both mechanisms seem possible. First, there is little doubt that under some conditions bubbles are exterior to the cell's surface and exert effects from that position. For example, Miller et al.[16] used a porous membrane to produce bubbles of a certain size; when insonated with spatial-peak intensities of 10–32 mW/cm² at 2.1 MHz blood platelets were observed to clump around the bubbles. This effect was obviously mediated by a form of stable cavitation. Under these conditions eddy currents are formed and "sweep" cells toward the bubbles. Such cavitation related effects can be mimicked by vibrating wires. With either a vibrating bubble or a vibrating wire in a fluid, strong microstreaming of the fluid around the vibrating object can create shear forces sufficient to shear (lyse) erythrocytes. Thus, it is clear that bubbles can affect cells from an extracellular position.

There is also some evidence that bubbles can penetrate cells, based on demonstrations that ultrasound can reduce cell viability and otherwise produce intracellular damage without inducing cell lysis. For example, Hedges and Leeman[17] exposed human lymphocytes to 1.5-MHz ultrasound at a (spatial average) intensity of 1.6 W/cm² and found evidence for damage to intracellular structures, the lysosomes, without producing lysis. As another example, Dooley et al. report that with insonated but intact cells thymine base damage occurs.[18] Also, Sacks et al.[19] have shown that insonated and intact multicell spheroid cells have agglomerated nuclei—that is, the nuclear and apparently not the cytoplasmic organization has been affected. Church et al.[20] have suggested that at least for a rotating tube system, a likely explanation for the observed effects is due to bubbles that "tunnel" into the cell; if the bubble is far from the membrane but near the nucleus when bubble implosion occurs, then the cell is not lysed and possibly becomes nonviable while remaining intact. If the implosion occurs near the membrane, lysis occurs. Alternatively, it is, of course, not necessary to assume that bubbles must be active inside a cell in order to account for intracellular damage. Nyborg and colleagues[21] have observed intracellular movements and disruptions in intact cells in arrangements where the cell membrane is vibrated locally by an external source such as a resonating bubble in intercellular space.

GENETIC EFFECTS

Has ultrasound been demonstrated to induce genetic effects in in vitro or related systems? No. There have been several attempts to determine if genetic effects are produced; see Chapter 6 of the present volume for a further discussion of this topic. The results are either negative or not confirmed for four broad categories of genetic or cytogenetic analysis: mutation, chromosome aberrations, nuclear agglomerations, and SCE. In general, there is no confirmed evidence that either mutations or chromosome aberrations are induced by ultrasound. There is reasonable agreement, particularly among scientists using plant systems, that ultrasound can induce nuclear agglomerations, a peculiar type of "welding" of the chromosome material, and this type of observations has been extended to multicell spheroids and has also been observed in lymphocytes and animal cells. It is not known exactly what an "agglomerated" nucleus is. Studies have shown that such a nucleus does not occur in a mitotic cell, and also that the incidence of such nuclei is relatively high soon after exposure to CW ultrasound and then rapidly diminishes. It appears that agglomerations do not persist in the cell population.

Sister Chromatid Exchange

A number of SCEs from a set of differentially stained human lymphocyte metaphase chromosomes (2N = 46) is illustrated in Figure 4.5. Each chromosome

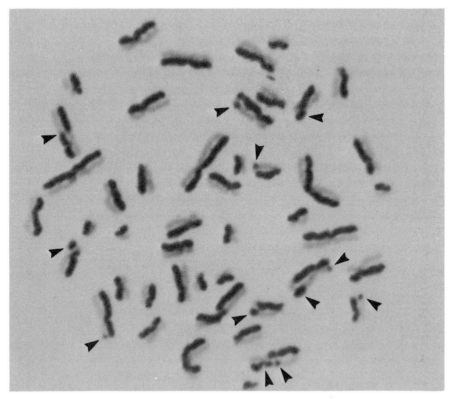

FIG. 4.5 Human lymphocytic harlequin metaphase chromosomes (2N = 46) showing sister chromatid exchanges (arrowheads). (Courtesy of Dr. A. Brulfert.)

at metaphase is composed of two chromatids (sisters). In order to determine whether or not the "sisters" have exchanged parts it is necessary to undertake a staining procedure which differentiates the sisters, that is, produces one darkly and one lightly stained chromatid per chromosome (i.e., a harlequin chromosome). With the production of differentiated or "harlequin" chromosomes, exchanges can be identified.

Whether or not ultrasound induces SCEs is not clear; the total literature in this area is summarized in Table 4.1. The intensities cited are "best estimates" and are usually as given by the authors. In some experiments the acoustic fields are complicated by reflection and/or other distortions and the experimental conditions are not well defined. There are several reports of positive effects (Liebeskind et al.,[22] Haupt et al.,[23] Barnett et al.,[24] Ehlinger et al.,[25]) and a large number of negative reports (Liebeskind et al.,[26] Morris et al.,[27] Wegner et al.,[28] Wegner and Meyenburg,[29] Barnett et al.,[30] Barrass et al.,[31] Au et al.,[32] Lundberg et al.,[33] Zheng et al.,[34] Miller et al.,[35] and Brulfert et al.[36, 37] The positive effects were not large in magnitude and it is possible that factors other than the exposure to ultrasound were contributing to the result, for example, some experiments were not scored blind. An increase in SCEs has been suggested to represent an increased genetic hazard,[38, 39] but this suggestion

TABLE 4.1 Reports dealing with sister chromatid exchange analyses and exposure to ultrasound[a]

Author	Cell Type	Type (In)	Mode	I_m (W/cm²)	I(SPTA)[b] (mW/cm²)	I(SPTA)[b] (W/cm²)	Results
Liebeskind et al.[26]	HeLa	Vitro	p	35.4	6.5–10	—	Negative
Liebeskind et al.[22]	Lymphocytes	Vitro	p	—	5.0	—	Positive
Haupt et al.[23]	Lymphocytes	Vitro	p	0.6	0.02	—	Positive
Morris et al.[27]	Lymphocytes	Vitro	CW	—	—	15–36	Negative
Zheng et al.[34]	Amniotic	Vivo	p	—	—	—	Negative
Au et al.[32]	Bone marrow	Vivo	CW	—	—	0.3–0.6[c]	Negative
Miller et al.[35]	Lymphocytes	Vitro	p	100	40	0	Negative
Brulfert et al.[36]	Lymphocytes	Vitro	p	2–200	0.3–30	—	Negative
			CW			2	Negative
Wegner et al.[28]	CHO (G₂)	Vitro	p	—	—	—	Negative
Lundberg et al.[33]	Amniotic	Vivo	p	—	—	—	Negative
Wegner and Meyenburg[29]	CHO (G₂, S)	Vitro	p	17	—	—	Negative
			CW	—	5.6(SATA)	—	Negative
Barnett et al.[30]	CHO	Vitro	p	—	—	0.1–45.	Negative
Barnett et al.[24]	CHO	Vitro	p	50–150	100–300	—	Negative
			p	650–2,500	—	1.3–5.0	Positive
Barrass et al.[31]	Fibroblasts	Vitro	CW	—	—	13.5	Negative
Ehlinger et al.[25]	Placentum	Vivo	p	—	—	—	Positive
Brulfert et al.[37]	Placentum	Vivo	p	0.25	—	—	Negative

Abbreviations: CHO, Chinese hamster ovary; p, pulsed; SATA, spatial-average temporal-average; other abbreviations as in text.

[a] Intensities cited are best estimates and are usually as given by the authors. In some experiments the acoustic fields are complicated by reflections and/or other distortions, and the experimental conditions are not well known. See Chapter 2 for definitions of SPTA and SATA intensities, and I_m.

[b] Except where indicated otherwise.

[c] Presumably spatial average; not clear over what area measurement refers to.

has not been established. Wolff and Carrano[40] have indicated that a wide variety of chemical and physical agents can induce SCEs, but neither their mechanism of formation or their genetic significance is understood.

MULTICELLULAR SPHEROIDS

It is now clear that ultrasound can induce through nonthermal mechanisms a variety of biological effects in in vitro systems. By contrast to research with in vitro single cells, however, whole tissues show few bioeffects at intensities characteristic of therapeutic applications, or at lower intensities, provided temperature is controlled. Multicellular spheroids, which are aggregates of in vitro cells, represent an organizational complexity intermediate between cells and tissues, and this may represent a "bridge" between single cell in vitro and multicellular in vivo systems. Multicell spheroids are a three-dimensional in vitro multicellular tissue culture system and provide the investigator with the option of analyzing the whole spheroid or its individual component cells for biological integrity.

Multicell spheroids have been exposed to ultrasound and assessed for growth. Conger et al.[41] reported a lack of effect on growth of whole spheroids exposed to 1 MHz ultrasound at exposures from 13 mW/cm² through 50 W/cm.² Their vessel was a plastic tube held stationary—that is, not rotated during insonation. Conversely, Sacks et al.[42] have also exposed multicell spheroids to 1-MHz ultrasound intensities of 1–5 W/cm² and showed that cell survival was affected in a dose-dependent relationship—the higher the dose the less survival. For the experiments of Sacks et al. the tube containing the spheroids was rotated during insonation. Additionally, it was also demonstrated that the effects induced in the spheroids were eliminated by increase in atmospheric pressure. Thus, the general conclusion from the single-cell in vitro results is also applicable to multicell spheroids; namely, that with the rotating tube system bioeffects are attributable to acoustic cavitation.

There are, however, some additional mechanistic insights which have been gained from research with spheroids. First, the fraction of spheroid surviving cells was higher than that of single cells—that is, the greater the number of cells per spheroid the more "resistant" it was to ultrasonically induced damage. Secondly, sonication of spheroids produced pycnotic cells, preferentially on the periphery. Thus, with death of the peripheral cells, those remaining "within" the spheroid would find their microenvironment richer with respect to oxygen and nutrients would be available for "repopulating" the spheroid. That the damage is primarily on the exterior of the spheroid suggests that cavitation and associated shear stresses occur in the fluid medium surrounding the spheroid and that damage from a cavitational mechanism is less likely within the multicellular organization. It is obvious that multicellularity per se results in some cellular shielding from potential ultrasonically induced cell damage.

Taken as a whole, the in vitro ultrasound literature indicates that ultrasound can induce a variety of biological effects. A number of investigations in this area have indicated that, in general, positive reports are correlated with stabilized bubbles. Acoustic cavitation appears to have played a major role in the induction of these effects.

ACKNOWLEDGEMENT

This study is based on work partially performed under contract no. DE-ACO2-76EV-3490, with the Department of Energy, The University of Rochester Department of Radiation Biology and Biophysics, and has been assigned report no. UR-3490–2255. Major support for this work was provided by United States Public Health Service Grant GM22680.

REFERENCES

1. Sacks P, Miller MW, Church CC: The exposure vessel as a factor in ultrasonically-induced mammalian cell lysis—I. A comparison of tube and chamber systems. Ultrasound Med Biol 8:289, 1982

2. Clarke PR, Hill CR: Biological action of ultrasound in relation to the cell cycle. Exp Cell Res 58:443, 1969

3. Church CC, Flynn HG, Miller MW, Sacks PG: The exposure vessel as a factor in ultrasonically-induced mammalian cell lysis—II. An explanation of the need to rotate exposure tubes. Ultrasound Med Biol 8:299, 1982

4. Ciaravino V, Miller MW, Carstensen EL: Pressure-mediated reduction of ultrasonically induced cell lysis. Radiat Res 88:209, 1981

5. Neppiras EA: Acoustic cavitation thresholds and cyclic process. Ultrasonics 18:201, 1980

6. Morton KI, Ter Haar G, Stratford IJ, Hill CR: The role of cavitation in the interaction of ultrasound with V79 Chinese hamster cells in vitro. Br J Cancer, 45:suppl. V, 147–150, 1982

7. Armour EP, Corry PM: Cytotoxic effects of ultrasound in vitro: dependence on gas content, frequency radical scavengers, and attachment. Radiat Res 89:369, 1982

8. Chater BV, Williams AR: Platelet aggregation induced in vitro by therapeutic ultrasound. Thrombos Haemostas 38:640, 1977

9. Fu YK, Miller MW, Kaufman GE, et al: Ultrasound lethality to synchronous and asynchronous Chinese hamster V-79 cells. Ultrasound Med Biol 6:39, 1980

10. Watmough DJ, Dendy PP, Eastwood LM, et al: The biophysical effects of therapeutic ultrasound on HeLa cells. Ultrasound Med Biol 3:205, 1977

11. Kaufman GE, Miller MW, Griffiths TD, et al: Lysis and viability of cultured mammalian cells exposed to 1 MHz ultrasound. Ultrasound Med Biol 3:21, 1977

12. Coakley WT, Hampton D, Dunn F: Qualitative relationships between ultrasonic cavitation and effects upon Amoebae at 1 MHz. J Acoust Soc Am 50:546, 1971

13. Moore JL, Coakley WT: Ultrasonic treatment of Chinese hamster cells at high intensities and long exposure times. Br J Radiol 50:46, 1977

14. Kremkau FW, Walker MM, Kaufmann JS, Spurr CL: Ultrasonic enhancement of cytotoxic effects of nitrogen mustard in mouse leukemia. J Acoust Soc Am, 55:suppl., 57, 1974

15. Chapman IV, MacNally NA, Tucker S: Ultrasound-induced changes in rates of influx and efflux of potassium ions in rat thymocytes in vitro. Ultrasound Med Biol 6:47, 1979

16. Miller DL, Nyborg WL, Whitcomb CC: Platelet aggregation induced by ultrasound under specialized conditions in vitro. Science 205:505, 1979

17. Hedges MJ, Leeman S: 1–5 MHz ultrasound irradiation of human lymphocytes. Int J Radiat Biol 35:301, 1979

18. Dooley DA, Sacks PG, Miller MW: Production of thymine base damage in ultrasound exposed EMT6 mouse mammary sarcoma cells. Radiat Res 97:71, 1984

19. Sacks PG, Miller MW: Ultrasonically induced nuclear aberrations in an *in vitro* multicellular tumor system. Br J Radiol 55:362, 1982

20. Church CC, Miller MW: On the kinetics and mechanics of ultrasonically-induced cell lysis produced by non-trapped bubbles in a rotating culture tube. Ultrasound Med Biol 9:385, 1983

21. Nyborg WL, Miller DL, Gershoy A: Physical consequences of ultrasound in plant tissues and other bio-systems, p. 277. In Michaelson S, Miller M, Magin R, Carstensen E (eds): Fundamental and Applied Aspects of Nonionizing Radiation. Plenum Press, New York, 1975

22. Liebeskind D, Bases R, Mendez F, et al: Sister chromatid exchanges in human lymphocytes after exposure to diagnostic ultrasound. Science 205:1273, 1979

23. Haupt M, Martin A, Simpson J, et al: Ultrasonic induction of sister chromatid exchanges in human lymphocytes. Hum Genet 59:221, 1981

24. Barnett SB, Bonin A, Mitchell G, et al: An investigation of the mutagenic potential of pulsed ultrasound. Br J Radiol 55:501, 1982

25. Ehlinger CA, Katayama KD, Roesler MR, Mattingly RF: Diagnostic ultrasound increases sister chromatid exchange; preliminary report. Wis Med J 80:21, 1981

26. Liebeskind D, Bases R, Koenisburg M, et al: Morphological changes in the surface characteristics of cultured cells after exposure to diagnostic ultrasound. Radiology 138:419, 1981

27. Morris SM, Palmer CG, Fry FJ, Johnson LK: Effect of ultrasound on human leucocytes. Sister chromatid exchange analysis. Ultrasound Med Biol 4:253, 1978

28. Wegner RD, Obe G, Meyenburg M: Has diagnostic ultrasound mutagenic effects? Hum Genet 56:95, 1980

29. Wegner R, Meyenburg M: The effects of diagnostic ultrasonography on the frequencies of sister chromatid exchanges in Chinese hamster cells and human lymphocytes. J Ultrasound Med 1:355, 1982

30. Barnett SB, Baker RSU, Barnstable S: Is pulsed ultrasound mutagenic? In Proceedings World Federation for Ultrasound in Medicine and Biology, Brighton, England, July 26–30, 1982

31. Barrass N, Ter Haar G, Casey G: The effect of ultrasound and hyperthermia on sister chromatid exchange and division kinetics of BHK21C13/A3 cells. Br J Cancer 45:187, 1982

32. Au W, Obergoenner N, Goldenthal K, et al: Sister-chromatid exchanges in mouse embryos after exposure to ultrasound *in utero*. Mutat Res 103:315, 1982

33. Lundberg M, Jermoniski L, Livingston G, et al: Failure to demonstrate an effect of *in vivo* diagnostic ultrasound on sister chromatid exchange frequency in amniotic fluid cells. Am J Med Genet 11:31, 1982

34. Zheng HZ, Mitter NS, Chudley AE: *In vivo* exposure to diagnostic ultrasound and *in vitro* assay of sister chromatid exchanges in cultured amniotic fluid cells. ICRS J Med Sci 9:491, 1981

35. Miller M, Wolff S, Filly R, et al: Absence of an effect of diagnostic ultrasound on sister chromatid exchange induction in human lymphocytes *in vitro*. Mutat Res 120:261, 1983

36. Brulfert A, Ciaravino V, Miller MW, Carstensen EL: Lack of ultrasound effect on *in vitro* human lymphocyte sister chromatid exchange. Ultrasound Med Biol 10:309, 1984

37. Brulfert A, Ciaravino V, Miller MW, et al: Diagnostic insonation of *extra utero* human placenta: no effect of lymphocytic sister chromatid exchange. Hum Genet 66:289, 1984

38. Perry PE, Evans HJ: Cytological detection of mutagen-carcinogen exposures by sister chromatid exchange. Nature 258:121, 1975

39. Kato H: Mechanisms of SCE's and their aberrations. Chromosomes 59:179, 1977

40. Wolff S, Carrano AV: Report of the workshop on the utility of sister chromatid exchange. Mutat Res 64:53, 1978
41. Conger AD, Ziskin MC, Wittels H: Ultrasonic effects on mammalian multicellular tumor spheroids. J Clin Ultrasound 9:167, 1981
42. Sacks PG, Miller MW, Sutherland RM: Response of multicell spheroids to 1-MHz ultrasonic irradiation: cavitation-related damage. Radiat Res 93:545, 1983

5 Effects of Ultrasound on Blood and the Circulation

A.R. WILLIAMS

The role of blood perfusion in the maintenance of tissue viability is so vital and ubiquitous that it is not possible to administer any diagnostic or therapeutic ultrasound exposure without also irradiating blood and the vessels which contain it. If ultrasound produces a relatively small change in the functional properties of the blood (e.g., an effect on leucocytes and their role in the immunologic protection of the animal) or in the ability of blood to flow through small vessels (i.e., any tendency to induce the blood to clot), it can exert a disproportionately large effect on the well-being of that animal.

Most of the experimental investigations of the bioeffects of ultrasound on blood performed to date have concentrated on one of five major topics. These are (1) the mechanical lysis of red blood cells in vitro, (2) effects on platelets and their role in the coagulation of blood, (3) functional effects on leucocytes and the reticuloendothelial system (4) chromosomal investigations in lymphocytes and related cells with a view to identifying possible genetic effects, and (5) vascular effects. Each of these topics will be reviewed separately. Before taking these up it is important to consider some of the mechanisms by which ultrasound acts on the cells. (See also Chapter 3.)

INTERACTION MECHANISMS

Temperature Elevation

Blood cells suspended in a relatively nonabsorbing medium like plasma are less likely to be affected by temperature rise than cells in compact or "solid" tissues because the absorbed heat can flow out of the small cells and into the cooler suspending medium.[1] This effect is accentuated if the cells are suspended in saline media in vitro. However, this cooling effect cannot happen if the cells are packed tightly together (as at very high hematocrits); in this case thermal effects may once again dominate as they appear to do in many soft tissue interactions. Bearing in mind the fact that blood is constantly in motion, so that the residence time of any given volume element of blood in the ultrasound beam is short, it is unlikely that the blood cells will experience a damaging temperature rise; an exception might occur when they are traversing the microvasculature of a heated tissue.

Cavitation

Cavitational activity, on the other hand, involves the pulsation of gas and vapor-filled bubbles (see Chapter 3). It is dependent upon many factors, including the intensity of the incident ultrasonic field, the presence of and number of appropriately sized gas bubbles, or the micronuclei from which they can grow, the geometry of the acoustic exposure situation, the composition and partial pressures of the various gases within the irradiated medium and the ambient temperature and pressure. A small gas bubble will dissolve completely unless it is protected from diffusion by some form of surface coat or skin, or is embedded within an irregularity on the surface of a solid body such as a dust particle.[2] Micronuclei are easily generated within liquid samples in vitro by mechanical handling, by placing them in contact with solid surfaces (especially if scratched or hydrophobic), by stirring,[3] or by exposing to certain types of ionizing radiation.[4]

When blood cells are exposed to ultrasound in vitro the conditions seen by the cells can be significantly different than when they are exposed in vivo, particularly if they have been resuspended in a saline medium at low hematocrit. Because of the factors mentioned above, thermal effects will have been minimized, whereas cavitational effects will have been maximized. The latter is especially true if some form of stirring or agitation system has been employed to maintain the cells as a homogenous suspension. Great care must therefore be exercized in the extrapolation of a bioeffect observed using isolated blood cells in vitro to the prediction of a potential hazard in vivo.

LYSIS OF RED BLOOD CELLS IN VITRO

Erythrocytes consist principally of membranes enclosing solutions of hemoglobin and are readily obtained as homogenous suspensions. They are readily lysed in a cavitating ultrasonic field. The lysis occurs at the lowest intensities in media containing preformed gas bubbles of a size close to the resonant dimensions for the particular ultrasonic driving frequency. In early work at kilohertz frequencies this situation was realized by drilling holes having diameters of the order of millimeters in the polished face of a metal velocity transformer.[5] More recently, stabilized gas bubbles having diameters of the order of microns (hence resonant at megahertz frequencies[6]) have been used; the bubbles were trapped in the pores of hydrophobic Nuclepore membranes.[7] When the use of these stabilized gas bubbles is combined with a sensitive technique capable of detecting the rupture of a small number of cells [e.g., a photometric technique employing firefly luciferin/luciferase for the detection of free adenosinetriphosphate (ATP)] then ultrasound-induced hemolysis can be observed (see Fig. 5.1) at spatial-peak intensities as low as 6 mW/cm² [continuous wave (CW), 1.6 MHz].[8, 9]

Gas bubbles tend to grow in a sound field. Hence bubbles that are too small to affect cells can be enlarged by the ultrasound itself until they are of an effective size. However, it requires a higher acoustic intensity to cause a small bubble, that is, a micronucleus, to grow into an effective bubble than is needed to drive a preexisting effective bubble into oscillation so that it can generate the streaming forces which modify or destroy biological tissues.[10] Consequently, any factor which generates micronuclei and/or assists the ultrasonic field in the initial stages of bubble growth will greatly enhance the amount of cavitational activity generated by any given ultrasonic intensity, if the latter is high enough. Williams[3] found evidence of this in experiments with CW ultrasound at a frequency of 0.75 MHz and intensity I_t (defined in Chapter 2) 0.6 W/cm² or 1.0 W/cm². He showed that the number of erythrocytes lysed by a given intensity of ultrasound increased as the rotational speed of a magnetic stirring bar contained within the sample chamber was increased. A similar enhancement of ultrasound-induced cavitational activity was also observed if the stirring bar was removed and the entire sample chamber oscillated at 50 Hz or was repeatedly struck by the corners of a rotating hexagonal metal bar.[3] It is presumed that the enhancement of cavitational activity by stirring results from both the generation of micronuclei by hydrodynamic nucleation, and the enhancement of bubble growth within the pressure gradients

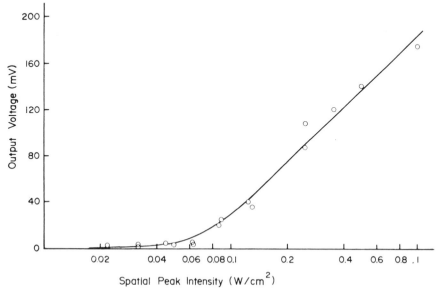

FIG. 5.1 Lysis of human erythrocytes (expressed as the voltage output from a photomultiplier tube) around gas bubbles stabilized within the pores of a Nuclepore membrane, as a function of the incident intensity of a 1.6-MH$_z$ beam of ultrasound.[8]

developed by the stirrer. If a stirred erythrocyte suspension is irradiated with pulsed ultrasound (0.75 MHz, 2 msec on and 8 msec off for 5 minutes) then cell lysis attributable to cavitational activity can be obtained at intensities (I_t) as low as about 2 mW/cm^2 (A. R. Williams, unpublished observations).

EFFECTS ON PLATELETS AND THEIR ROLE IN THE COAGULATION OF BLOOD

Platelets are blood-borne anucleate cell fragments which can be stimulated by a wide range of chemical and physical factors including collagen, adenosine diphosphate (ADP), electrical current, mechanical trauma and hydrodynamic shear stress. Their first response to a suprathreshold stimulus is to undergo a shape change (a disc-to-echinocyte transition) and become "sticky" so that they attach themselves to any available solid surface (adhesion) or to each other (aggregation). This shape change is usually followed by the "release reaction" which involves the active expulsion of the contents of the platelet's secretory granules and vacuoles. These contents can be roughly divided into three classes of chemicals, which are: (1) vasoactive substances such as histamine and serotonin which result in a transient vasoconstriction, (2) platelet-aggregating factors including ADP which cause more platelets to attach themselves to the growing platelet thrombus, and (3) coagulation factors (including platelet factor 3) which initiate and accelerate the plasma coagulation system resulting in the rapid conversion of fibrinogen to fibrin and the eventual formation of a true red blood clot.[11]

Numerous diverse techniques have been employed to determine the effects of ultrasonic energy on platelets and their physiological role. Experiments have been carried out, both in vitro and in vivo, at a low ultrasonic frequency (about 20 kHz), using models to simulate the small-scale streaming fields developed around oscillating gas bubbles. The object of these studies was to see if cavitation-induced forces could initiate blood coagulation in vitro and in vivo. Other investigations were carried out in the megahertz frequency range characteristic of therapeutic ultrasound; in vitro experiments dealt with platelets and the blood coagulation system, while the in vivo experiments included tests for changes in the blood of living animals and human volunteers.

The Effects of Acoustic Microstreaming Fields on Platelets

Small gas bubbles are difficult to control (unless they are stabilized within holes in solid bodies) because they tend to dissolve spontaneously or, in an ultrasound field, to be driven out of the region of interest by radiation pressure forces. However, research on their effects can be carried out by use of models. The acoustic microsteaming fields generated around the hemispherical tips of small metal wires or probes oscillating at ultrasonic frequencies while immersed in a liquid[12, 13] are similar to those generated by gas bubbles oscillating in a stable manner, especially if the bubbles are in contact with a solid surface.[14] These models of stable cavitational activity are less prone to artifact and are usually more amenable to quantification than acoustic microstreaming fields induced by gas bubbles.

Nyborg[15] developed an approximate theory which predicted that the magnitude of the hydrodynamic shear stresses generated within these acoustic microstreaming fields should increase as the square of the displacement amplitude of the oscillating body. Williams[16] exposed functionally inert human platelets containing radioactively labeled serotonin to the acoustic microstreaming field generated around a 250-μm-diameter steel or tungsten wire oscillating in a transverse mode at 20 kHz and observed that, as had been hypothesized, the amount of serotinin released increased in a linear manner when plotted against the square of the wire displacement amplitude. These experiments strongly indicate that it is the acoustic microstreaming field generated around wires or gas bubbles which disrupts platelets. Comparison with results of similar experiments with erythrocytes shows that platelets are about 10 times more fragile than erythrocytes.[12, 16]

If a small blood vessel is exposed in an anesthetized animal, these metal wires or probes can be pressed against the outside of the vessel wall so as to make an indentation similar to that made by pushing a finger into an air or water-filled balloon. The mechanical coupling between the wire and the vessel wall is so efficient that the indented portion of the vessel wall can be driven to oscillate at the same ultrasonic frequency and at the same displacement amplitude as the metal wire.[17, 18] When transilluminated and viewed under the microscope it can be seen that the oscillating portion of the vessel wall generates an acoustic microstreaming field within the intact blood vessel (Fig. 5.2) and that a variety of displacement-amplitude-dependent biological effects can be observed.

At the lowest displacement amplitudes used, the flowing blood could be seen to be deflected from its normal streamlines and to form twin vortices at the point of contact with the wire tip. No damage to the blood cells or the endothelium could be detected although slightly higher displacement amplitudes resulted in the adhesion of platelets having partially disrupted membranes to the apparently normal endothelium.[17, 18] At higher displacement amplitudes the twin vortices grow to fill the lumen of the small vessels and gelatinous aggregates of platelets are observed to form in the center of the vortices (Fig. 5.2) and to embolize downstream where they adhere to the vessel wall if they touch it. At even higher displacement amplitudes the platelet aggregates emerge as a continuous stream from the microstreaming vortices and create a thrombus downstream (due to the formation of fibrin) where it may occlude the blood vessel.[17, 18]

Thus, platelets are easily disrupted and/or stimulated to participate in the formation of a thrombus both in vitro and in vivo by acoustic microstreaming fields. These observations suggest that similar fields generated around oscillating gas bubbles (if they were to occur in blood during ultrasound exposure in vivo) could pose a potential thrombogenic hazard.

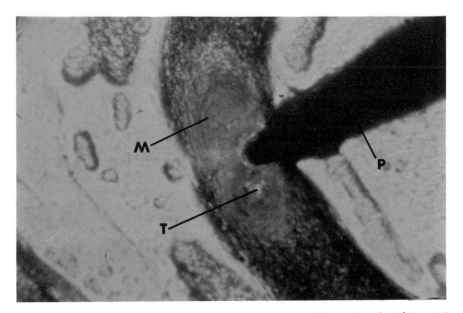

FIG. 5.2 Photomicrograph of the microstreaming vortices (M) produced within a 200-μm-diameter mouse mesenteric blood vessel in vivo by the external application of a metal probe (P) oscillating at 85 kHz.[18] A platelet thrombus (T) can be seen within one of the microstreaming vortices.

In Vitro Studies at Megahertz Frequencies

A number of investigations has been carried out on platelets in anticoagulated whole blood or in platelet-rich plasma (PRP, i.e., anticoagulated blood from which the erythrocytes and most of the leukocytes have been removed by centrifugation), exposed to ultrasound in vitro under free-field exposure conditions, that is, conditions where standing waves are avoided. Williams et al.[19] demonstrated that 5-min exposures of citrated PRP to 1-MHz CW ultrasound at spatial-peak intensities of 0.18 W/cm² and higher resulted in a time-dependent decrease in the "recalcification time" (the time taken to form macroscopic strands of fibrin following the addition of enough calcium ions to overcome the effects of the anticoagulant). This increased tendency of the blood to clot was associated with numerous morphologic changes in the structure of the clot as seen by electron microscopy. Sonicated PRP gave larger, less rigid clots containing multivacuolated cells and numerous platelet fragments which were not present in control samples.[20] These changes in recalcification time and clot morphology could be duplicated by incubating control PRP with small quantities of homogenized PRP prior to recalcification.[20]

Chater and Williams[21] devised a free-field ultrasound exposure apparatus whereby the rate and extent of platelet aggregation could be measured while the samples were being exposed to 0.75 MHz CW ultrasound. They found that ultrasound exposure alone could induce human platelets in citrated PRP to aggregate.[21] At any given ultrasonic frequency there was an apparent "threshold" intensity below which the sample did not aggregate (this was typically about 0.6–0.8 W/cm^2 (I_t). At any given suprathreshold intensity, the extent of aggregation decreased as the ultrasonic frequency was increased.[21] For any one human donor the amount of aggregation produced by a given suprathreshold intensity was remarkably constant. However, PRP from different donors sometimes exhibited wide variations in the rate and extent of aggregation induced by the same intensity of ultrasound. This variability was traced to the different inherent sensitivities of the platelets from different donors to physiologically induced aggregation. Those samples which required low concentrations of ADP to induce aggregation required a lower "threshold" intensity of ultrasound whereas those samples requiring high concentrations of ADP before aggregating had higher "threshold" intensity values.[21]

These measurements on ultrasound-induced aggregation together with the recalcification time data outlined above strongly suggested that ultrasound was exerting its effects by disrupting a small proportion of the platelet population (possibly via a cavitational mechanism) and it was the materials released from the disrupted platelets which were responsible for the observed changes. This hypothesis is supported by the observation that PRP samples irradiated with "subthreshold" intensities of ultrasound (i.e., intensities less than the value required to induce spontaneous aggregation) were refractory (i.e., less sensitive to low concentrations of an aggregating agent) when challenged with more ADP.[21] This is analogous to the observation that two subthreshold doses of ADP given about 10 min apart do not result in platelet aggregation even though the final ADP concentration is greater than the threshold value for a single administration of ADP.

Additional information supporting this hypothesis came from measurements of the rate of liberation of β-thromboglobulin (β-TG), a platelet-specific protein of unknown function which is contained within the platelet α-granules and is liberated when they undergo the release reaction or are disrupted.[22, 23]

All of the above results indicate that some form of cavitational activity is being generated at "suprathreshold" intensities of ultrasound which subsequently disrupts a small proportion of the platelet population (and also some of the erythrocyte population if they are also present). When enough cells have been disrupted, the materials liberated from these cells, especially ADP, will induce other undamaged functional platelets to undergo their normal release reaction; these liberate β-TG and more ADP, and also aggregate, thus initiating a self-perpetuating cycle which continues as long as there are normal platelets present.

As in the case of erythrocytes, the ultrasonic intensity needed to initiate platelet aggregation is greatly reduced if the irradiated medium is stirred or agitated or supplied with preformed gas bubbles of resonant size stabilized within the pores of Nuclepore membranes. Miller et al.[24] showed that human platelets in citrated PRP formed aggregates in the vicinity of the gas-filled

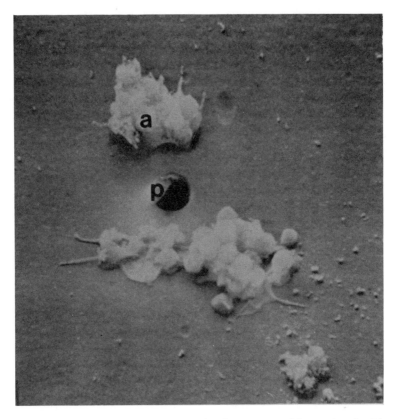

FIG. 5.3 Scanning electron photomicrograph of aggregates (a) associated with a pore (p) after exposure to ultrasound generated by a Doppler ultrasound device used in medicine (pore diameter, 4.5 μm).[24]

pores at spatial-peak intensities of only 16–32 mW/cm^2 (CW, 2.1 MHz). It was then shown that, as expected, the platelets could be induced to aggregate by the ultrasonic field emitted by a common Doppler diagnostic instrument used for the detection of the foetal heart[24] (see Fig. 5.3). Some of these platelets have been disrupted or induced to undergo the release reaction as demonstrated by the luciferase/luciferin enzyme system for the detection of free ATP.[25]

In Vivo Studies at Megahertz Frequencies

The investigations outlined above indicate that platelet damage in vitro is primarily a result of some form of cavitational activity; hence it is reasonable to assume that similar effects would occur if cavitational activity were to be induced within the intact vascular system in vivo. Preliminary in vivo investigations using megahertz frequencies of ultrasound were inconclusive in that Zarod and Williams[26] found occasional small aggregates of platelets trapped within the microcirculation of the external ear of a guinea pig after its main blood supply vessel (the central ear artery) had been subjected to 1 W/cm² (I_t) of 0.75-MHz pulsed and 3-MHz CW ultrasound. However, subsequent investigations demonstrated significant temperature elevations under these exposure conditions; it now seems that the platelet aggregates may have been initiated by tissue thromboplastins released from thermally damaged endothelium.

In a subsequent series of investigations, butterfly cannulae were inserted into the anticubital veins of health adult human volunteers and a 0.75-MHz transducer was positioned about 2.5 cm upstream of the puncture site.[27] Blood samples were collected before, during, and after the transducer had been activated at the highest intensity that the volunteers would tolerate (typically 0.35–0.5 W/cm² I_t, CW). There was no detectable elevation in the plasma levels of β-TG in the samples collected while the ultrasound was being administered.[27] In an attempt to subject blood in vivo to higher intensities of ultrasound we used a rabbit model. Rabbit platelets are loaded with histamine which is liberated when they undergo the release reaction or are disrupted. When rabbit blood vessels were exposed to intensities (I_t) as high as 17.4 W/cm² no increase in the level of plasma histamine or free hemoglobin could be detected.[28]

Contradictory results were reported by Wong and Watmough[29] who found evidence of intravascular hemolysis after they irradiated the beating hearts of anesthetized mice for 5 minutes with 0.7 to 2 W/cm² [spatial-average temporal-average (SATA), CW] of 0.75-MHz CW ultrasound. One of the major differences between this exposure situation and the ones employed above, besides the size of the animal investigated, is that here the blood is being violently agitated within the heart while it is being exposed to the ultrasound. It is possible that these turbulent rheologic conditions could generate cavitation nuclei and/or assist the growth of nuclei to form bubbles[3] so that cavitational activity could occur in vivo at ultrasonic intensities which are known to be ineffective in nonturbulent blood. This possibility is currently under investigation in several laboratories but preliminary results have not been able to demonstrate the occurrence of intravascular cavitation at therapeutic intensities of ultrasound in rabbits or dogs even when the beating heart is irradiated.[30]

Lunan et al.[31] exposed anesthetized mice to whole-body CW ultrasonic irradiation for 5 min at 2 MHz at a spatial-average intensity of 1 W/cm² in a 37°C water bath. Four hours following the exposure, platelets were found to aggregate less efficiently than those from control animals. It is not known if this reflects a direct effect of ultrasound on the platelets (i.e. a possible refractory phase following a "subthreshold" stimulation) or a general systemic effect resulting from the release of substances such as prostaglandins into the animal's bloodstream.

Controversial results were reported by Yaroniene[32] who subjected the hearts of rabbits for 2 weeks or 1 month to 2-MHz ultrasound (either CW at intensity 10 mW/cm², I_t, or in pulses of duration 4 μsec, repetition frequency 1 kHz, and intensity 0.4 mW/cm², I_t) from a portable ultrasonic device which was strapped to the animal's body. Histologic investigation showed changes in the chest muscles, myocardium, and liver: the reported changes included capillary expansion, microthrombus formation, and erythrocyte aggregation.[32] Details of the experiments are not available.

Ultrasonic Contrast Agents

One potential health hazard involving the possible interaction between ultrasound and platelets which has not yet been investigated in detail concerns the role of ultrasonic contrast agents. Most of these agents function by introducing large numbers of micron-sized gas bubbles into the bloodstream so as to efficiently scatter the interrogating ultrasound beam and so generate strong echoes.[33] Some of these bubbles are close to the resonant dimensions for the ultrasound frequencies being employed. Thus, the use of ultrasonic contrast agents simulates the in vitro experiments using gas bubbles of resonant dimensions stabilized within the pores of hydrophobic Nuclepore membranes. These in vitro gas bubbles can induce platelet aggregation at diagnostic intensity levels[7] and so it is not unreasonable to presume that the gas bubbles introduced during contrast echocardiography may be capable of producing similar effects. This topic is currently under investigation. The use of nongaseous contrast agents, such as collagen microspheres, is also being explored; these agents would presumably not present potential for cavitation effects.

Turbulent Blood Flow

Experimental evidence indicates that diagnostic and therapeutic intensities of ultrasound do not appear to damage platelets in vivo or initiate blood coagulation, provided that excessive temperature elevations are avoided. However, there are several possibilities which have not been fully explored; one is that turbulent blood flow may aid in the induction of acoustically driven cavitation. Because of this uncertainty it would therefore be prudent not to expose the beating heart of the adult or fetus to high therapeutic intensities of ultrasound. Another possibility is that ultrasound contrast agents might cause thrombogenic effects, especially in combination with other factors, such as turbulent flow fields and/or the development of standing waves.

FUNCTIONAL CHANGES IN LEUCOCYTES AND THE RETICULOENDOTHELIAL SYSTEM

Crowell et al.[34] subjected white-cell-enriched canine plasma to the acoustic microstreaming field generated around a tungsten wire oscillating transversely at 20 kHz. They observed cell lysis at wire displacement amplitudes greater than 8 μm. At amplitudes significantly less than the value required to disrupt the cells, they measured changes in phagocytic and bacteriocidal indexes and metabolic activities. Visual observation of the number of bacteria engulfed by (and/or adhering to the surface of) the polymorphonuclear neutrophilic leucocytes showed that the average cell's phagocytic index increased with increasing wire displacement amplitude up to about 7 μm and thereafter decreased with still larger displacement amplitudes. Conversely, the number of bacteria killed by each leucocyte (i.e., its relative bactericidal capacity) declined progressively with increasing displacement amplitude suggesting that more bacteria may be attached to the outside of sheared cells rather than being engulfed by them.[34] This increased adhesion might be due to changes in the distribution of charges on the cell surface resulting from exposure to the microstreaming field as has been shown for human erythrocytes exposed to ultrasound[35, 36] at megahertz frequencies.

Other authors have observed similar functional changes after leucocytes had been exposed to ultrasound in vitro at frequencies in the lower megahertz range. For example, Fung et al.[37] report a decrease in the rate of uptake of labeled thymidine by human lymphocytes after they had been exposed to ultrasound at diagnostic frequencies and intensities.

Anderson and Barrett[38] irradiated the splenic area of mice for 5 minutes with pulsed 2-MHz ultrasound [spatial-peak temporal-average (SPTA) intensity 8.9 mW/cm^2] and evaluated the ability of test and control animals to raise antibodies against an intraperitoneal injection of sheep erythrocytes. Their results apparently show a decrease, or "desensitization," of the immune response in the irradiated animals. However, the magnitude of this decrease was small compared with the capacity of the immune system to respond to a potentially serious immunologic challenge, and two independent laboratories have been unable to confirm these findings.[39]

Ford et al.[40] have developed a sensitive technique for quantifying an animal's immunologic competence by measuring the results of the competition between an animal's lymphocytes and foreign lymphocytes in vivo. A known number of foreign lymphocytes are injected into the hind foot pads of mice and permitted to migrate through the lymphatic system to the popliteal lymph nodes. Here, the host lymphocytes are attracted and proliferate and usually destroy the invaders. The resulting weight gain of the lymph node is measured (it can increase by a factor of up to 70-fold). It was found that neither of the following procedures produced a measureable change in node weight: (1) ultrasonic irradiation of the invading lymphocytes in vitro before injection; (2) ultrasonic irradiation of one of an animal's popliteal lymph nodes in vivo after both hind limbs had been injected with the same number of foreign cells. For both procedures the ultrasound was continuous at a frequency of 3 MHz and intensity of 0.8 W/cm^2, I_t.[41]

Another function associated with the immunologic system is the mechanism whereby cell debris and solid particles are cleared from the blood by the cells of the reticuloendothelial system, which are found mainly within the liver, lungs, spleen, bone marrow and lymphoid tissue. In an experiment designed to test the response of this immune function to ultrasound, colloidal sulfur particles radiolabeled with technetium[99m] were injected in saline suspension into an anesthetized rat via a tail vein. In the absence of ultrasound these particles were found to be cleared from the blood at a characteristic exponential rate.[42] Irradiation of the umbilical area with 0.75-MHz CW ultrasound for 5 minutes at intensities (I_t) greater than about 0.8 W/cm² decreased the rate at which the sulfur colloid was removed from the blood. The magnitude of this reversible change increased with increasing intensity or exposure time.[44] A novel observation was that isolated lymphocytes irradiated with ultrasound in vitro and reinjected via the tail vein before the administration of the colloidal sulfur, also resulted in a similar decrease in the rate of removal of colloid whereas the reinjection of control lymphocytes did not.[43]

Thus in vivo ultrasonic irradiation at intensities characteristic of therapeutic ultrasound has been shown to change the functional behavior of leucocytes and the reticuloendothelial system. The observed changes are small compared with the changes normally seen in response to infections and so it does not appear that ultrasonic irradiation poses a significant threat to health based upon the evidence currently available.

CHROMOSOMAL CHANGES IN LYMPHOCYTES

This topic is taken up in detail in Chapters 4 and 6 of this volume, and will be discussed only briefly here. The mutagenic capacity of chemical substances or ionizing radiations is frequently assessed by their ability to produce chromosomal abnormalities[44] (broken or abnormal chromosomes or perhaps even changes in the frequency of sister chromatid exchange) in suspensions of human lymphocytes in culture. Therefore, the reports by Macintosh and Davey[45, 46] that the ultrasonic field emitted by a commercially available diagnostic device increased the incidence of chromosomal aberrations in cultured human lymphocytes, caused great concern and initiated an intensive series of investigations to duplicate these investigations. While a few of the subsequent reports apparently confirmed these initial observations, the vast majority indicated that neither diagnostic nor therapeutic intensities of MHz ultrasound had any effect upon the incidence of chromosome abnormalities (see Chapter 6 for details). A major criticism of the original reports by Macintosh and Davey[45, 46] was that an observer bias could have been introduced during the scoring of the spread chromosomes. In a subsequent article when the original chromosome spreads were rescored in a double-blind manner, no increase in chromosome abnormalities could be detected.[47]

Sister chromatid exchange (SCE) has been advocated as a more sensitive technique for the assessment of nuclear damage,[48] although Gebhart[44] has pointed out that the molecular mechanisms responsible for the formation of SCEs and chromosome breaks are different. Reports that diagnostic ultrasound, applied to human lymphocytes, caused an increased rate of SCE formation, led to concern among the medical community. The numerous attempts (mostly unsuccessful) to confirm these findings are discussed in detail in Chapters 4 and 6.

There are sufficient ambiguities and potential sources of artefact in the evidence currently available that it is reasonable to conclude that ultrasound does not appear to modify the nuclear material within lymphocytes. In fact, the interaction mechanisms of ionizing radiation and ultrasound with biological tissues are so different that it would be remarkable if they exerted the same biological effects. While it is possible that ultrasound may result in changes such as an increased incidence of SCE, it is highly probable that these effects are caused by direct mechanical damage to the cells resulting from some form of cavitational activity and not by chemical modification of the DNA. Chemical modification of DNA could perhaps occur as a result of free radicals generated in vivo by transient cavitation, but the probability of this occurring is extremely low as the cells are most likely to be disrupted by the cavitation before they can be chemically modified. Even if the free radicals were able to survive long enough to encounter an intact cell, they would most probably interact with membrane or cytoplasmic constituents long before they could enter the nucleus. Ionizing radiation can generate its free radicals directly within the nucleus of an intact cell.

EFFECTS ON THE VASCULAR SYSTEM

The ultrasonic exposure conditions are markedly different for a tissue or organ subjected to an acoustic field having a strong standing-wave component as compared with the organ subjected to an ultrasound beam of the same incident intensity in the absence of a reflected wave. Dyson et al.[49] have shown that a standing wave results in the reversible accumulation of the blood cells in discrete bands, with interband spacing equal to one half wavelength of the compressional wave (Fig. 5.4). There is no single "threshold" intensity for the production of this effect, called blood cell stasis, since it depends upon the ultrasonic frequency, the magnitude of the standing-wave component, the animal's blood pressure, the velocity of blood flow within that vessel, and the dimensions and orientation of the vessel relative to the axis of the ultrasound beam, as well as the difference in density between the blood cells and the surrounding plasma. Under laboratory conditions this effect cannot usually be observed at intensities less than about 0.5 W/cm^2 (spatial-peak) at 3 MHz (CW), and can be avoided at even higher intensities if the irradiating transducer is kept moving or if short pulses of ultrasound are used. Blood cell stasis prevents the normal circulation of erythrocytes and so tissue anoxia may result if stasis is maintained for prolonged periods.

Another major change in the acoustic exposure conditions brought about by the development of a standing-wave field is the enhancement of the development of cavitational activity. Microbubbles smaller than resonant size are driven to the antinodes of pressure amplitude where they may grow to a resonant size. It is presumably these oscillating bubbles which were responsible for the mechanical disruption of the vascular endothelium reported by ter Haar et al.[50] (Fig. 5.5) and the consolidation of the red cell band with fibrin to form an irreversible "plug" which did not break down when the acoustic field was turned off.

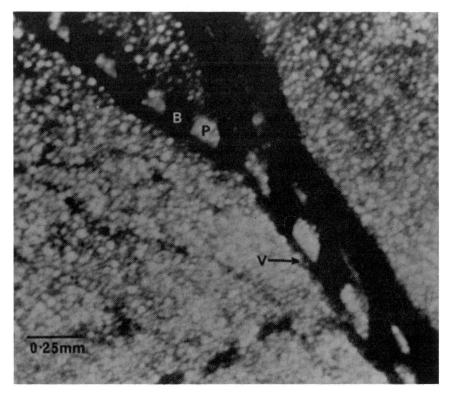

FIG. 5.4 Surface view of the area vasculosa showing blood cell stasis. The cell bands (B) in the vein (V) are at half-wavelength intervals, and are separated by pale areas of plasma (P).[50]

Lizzi et al.[51] reported a novel reversible bioeffect in that the retinal blood supply of an albino rabbit was seen to blanch within the focal volume of a focused bowl transducer when it was subjected to an intensity-time combination just below the level required to produce a (thermal) chorioretinal lesion. This blanched region disappeared when the ultrasound was turned off. It is not known if this transient blanching is due to microvascular constriction (i.e., direct neural or neuromuscular stimulation by the ultrasound) or is a mechanical effect resulting from the compression of the nutrient capillaries by the radiation pressure forces emanating from the transducer.

A similar ultrasound-induced transient vasoconstriction within the microvasculature of the external ear of a guinea pig was observed by Zarod and Williams (unpublished observations). However, the effect was highly variable in its occurrence and was only observed under conditions where thermal damage to the pinna would be expected.

With the possible exception of prolonged blood-cell stasis, which might

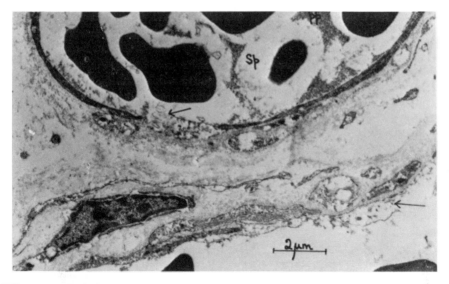

FIG. 5.5 Endothelial cell damage in two adjacent blood vessels (delayed excision). In some regions (arrowed) the endothelium is completely disrupted. The spaces (Sp) between the precipitated plasma (PP) and the erythrocytes (ER) indicate considerable cell shrinkage during processing.[51]

occur during an application of ultrasound therapy, it is unlikely that effects induced by ultrasound upon the vascular system will prove to be a hazard of concern in medical applications.

REFERENCES

1. Love LA, Kremkau FW: Intracellular temperature distribution produced by ultrasound. J Acoust Soc Am 67:1045, 1980
2. Crum LA: Tensile strength of water. Nature 278:148, 1979
3. Williams AR: Absence of meaningful thresholds for bioeffect studies on cell suspensions *in vivo*. Br J Cancer 56:192, 1982
4. Messino D, Sette D, Wanderlingh F: Statistical approach to ultrasonic cavitation. J Acoust Soc Am 35:1575, 1963
5. Hughes DE, Nyborg WL: Cell disruption by ultrasound. Science 138:108, 1962
6. Miller DL: Experimental investigation of the response of gas-filled micropores to ultrasound. J Acoust Soc Am 71:471, 1982
7. Miller DL, Nyborg WL, Whitcomb CC: Platelet aggregation induced by ultrasound under specialized conditions *in vitro*. Science 205:505, 1979
8. Williams AR, Miller DL: Photometric detection of ATP release from human erythrocytes exposed to ultrasonically activated gas-filled pores. Ultrasound Med Biol 6:251, 1980
9. Miller DL, Williams AR: Further investigations of ATP release from human erythrocytes exposed to ultrasonically activated gas-filled pores. Ultrasound Med Biol 9:297, 1983
10. Nyborg WL: Physical Mechanisms for Biological Effects of Ultrasound. Department of Health, Education and Welfare Publication (FDA) 78–8062, Rockville, Maryland, 1978

11. Thomas D: Haemostasis. Br Med Bull 33:183, 1977

12. Williams AR, Hughes DE, Nyborg WL: Haemolysis near a transversely oscillating wire. Science 169:871, 1970

13. Holtzmark J, Johnsen I, Sikkeland T, Skavlem S: Boundary layer flow near a cylindrical obstacle in an oscillating incompressible fluid. J Acoust Soc Am 26:26, 1954

14. Rooney JA: Hemolysis near an ultrasonically pulsating gas bubble. Science 169:869, 1970

15. Nyborg WL: Acoustic streaming. p. 265. In Mason WP (ed): Physical Acoustics. Vol. 2B. Academic Press, New York, 1965

16. Williams AR: Release of serotonin from human platelets by acoustic microstreaming. J Acoust Soc Am 56:1640, 1974

17. Williams AR: Intravascular mural thrombi produced by acoustic microstreaming. Ultrasound Med Biol 3:191, 1977

18. Williams AR: *In vivo* thrombogenesis. In Gross DR, Hwang NHC (eds): The Rheology of Blood, Blood Vessels and Associated Tissues. Sijhoff and Noordhoff, The Netherlands, 1981

19. Williams AR, O'Brien WD, Coller BS: Exposure to ultrasound decreases the recalcification time of platelet rich plasma. Ultrasound Med Biol 2:113, 1976

20. Williams AR, Sykes SM, O'Brien WD: Ultrasonic exposure modifies platelet morphology and function *in vitro*. Ultrasound Med Biol 2:311, 1976

21. Chater BV, Williams AR: Platelet aggregation induced *in vitro* by therapeutic ultrasound. Thrombos Haemostas 38:640, 1977

22. Ludlam CA, Moore S, Bolton AE, et al: The release of human platelet-specific protein measured by a radioimmunoassay. Thrombos Res 6:543, 1975

23. Williams AR, Chater BV, Allen KA, et al: Release of β-thromboglobulin from human platelets by therapeutic intensities of ultrasound. Br J Haematol 40:133, 1978

24. Miller DL, Nyborg WL, Whitcomb CC: *In vitro* clumping of platelets exposed to low intensity ultrasound. P. 45. In White DN, Lyons EA (eds): Ultrasound in Medicine. Vol. 4. Plenum Press, New York, 1978

25. Miller DL, Williams AR, Nyborg WL: Photochemical detection of platelet damage induced by low intensity ultrasound. Reflections 5:193, 1979

26. Zarod AP. Williams AR: Platelet aggregation *in vivo* by therapeutic ultrasound. Lancet 2:1266, 1977

27. Williams AR, Chater BV, Allen KA, Sanderson JH: The use of -thromboglobulin to detect platelet damage by therapeutic ultrasound *in vivo*. J Clin Ultrasound 9:145, 1981

28. Chater BV, Williams AR: Absence of platelet damage *in vivo* following the exposure of non-turbulent blood to therapeutic ultrasound. Ultrasound Med Biol 8:85, 1982

29. Wong YS, Watmough DJ: Haemolysis of red blood cells *in vitro* and *in vivo* caused by therapeutic ultrasound at 0.75 MHz. p. 179. In Millner R, Rosenfeld E, Cobet U (eds): Ultrasound Interactions in Biology and Medicine. Plenum Press, New York, 1983

30. Gross DR, Miller DL, Williams AR: A search for ultrasonic cavitation within the canine cardiovascular system. Ultrasound in Med Biol (in press)

31. Lunan KD, Wen AC, Barfod ET, et al: Decreased aggregation of mouse platelets after *in vivo* exposure to ultrasound. Thrombos Haemos 40:568, 1979

32. Yaroniene G: Response of biological systems to low-intensity ultrasonic waves. In Filipczynski L, Zieniuk JK (eds): Proceedings of the Second Congress of the Federation of Acoustical Societies of Europe, Vol. 2. Warsaw, 1972

33. Roelandt J: Contrast echocardiography. Ultrasound Med Biol 8:471, 1982

34. Crowell JA, Kusserow BK, Nyborg WL: Functional changes in white blood cells after microsonation. Ultrasound Med Biol 3:185, 1977

35. Hrazdira I: Cellular effects of ultrasound. Proceedings 4th Euorpean Conference Ultrasound in Medicine Biology, Dubrovnik, Yugoslavia, May 18–22, 1981

36. Pinamonti S, Mazzeo V, Pedrielli F, et al: Functional changes in human erythrocytes caused by pulsed ultrasound *in vitro*. Proceedings 4th European Conference Ultrasound in Medicine and Biology, Dubrovnik, Yugoslavia, May 18–22, 1981 cytes exposed to ultrasound. Ultrasound Med Biol 1980

37. Fung H, Cheung K, Lyons EA, Kay NE: The effect of low dose ultrasound on human peripheral lymphocyte function *in vitro*. P. 583. In White DN, Lyons EA (eds): Ultrasound in Medicine. Vol. 4. Plenum Press, New York, 1978

38. Anderson DW, Barrett JT: Ultrasound: a new immunosuppressant. Clin Immunol Pathol 14:18, 1979

39. Child SZ, Hare JD, Carstensen EL, et al: Test for the effects of diagnostic levels of ultrasound on the immune response of mice. Clin Immunol Immunopathol 18:299, 1981

40. Ford WL, Burr W, Simonsen M: A lymph node weight assay for the graft-versus-host activity of rat lymphoid cells. Transplantation 10:258, 1970

41. Williams AR, Saad AH, Ford WL: In preparation

42. Saad AH, Williams AR: Effects of therapeutic ultrasound on clearance rate of blood borne colloidal particles *in vivo*. Br J Cancer 45:202, 1982

43. Saad AH, Williams AR: Therapeutic ultrasound and the mononuclear phagocyte system— effects *in vivo* and possible mechanisms. In preparation

44. Gebhart E: Sister chromatid exchange (SCE) and structural chromosome aberration in mutagenicity testing. Hum Genet 58:235, 1981

45. Macintosh IJC, Davey DA: Chromosome aberrations induced by an ultrasonic foetal pulse detector. Br Med J 4:92, 1970

46. Macintosh IJC, Davey DA: Relationship between intensity of ultrasound and induction of chromosome aberrations. Br J Radiol 45:320, 1972

47. Macintosh IJC, Brown RC, Coakley WT: Ultrasound and *in vitro* chromosome aberrations. Br J Radiol 48:230, 1975

48. Carrano AV, Thompson LH, Lindl PA, Minkler JL: Sister chromatid exchange as an indicator of mutagenesis. Nature 271:551, 1978

49. Dyson M, Pond JB, Woodward B, Broadbent J: The production of blood cell stasis and endothelial damage in the blood vessels of chick embryos treated with ultrasound in a stationary wave field. Ultrasound Med Biol 1:133, 1974

50. ter Haar G, Dyson M, Smith SP: Ultrastructural changes in the mouse uterus brought about by ultrasonic irradiation at therapeutic intensities in standing wave fields. Ultrasound Med Biol 5:167, 1979

51. Lizzi FL, Coleman DJ, Driller J et al: Experimental ultrasonically induced lesions in the retina, choroid and sclera. Invest Ophthalmol Vis Sci 17:350, 1978

6 Investigations into Genetic and Inherited Changes Produced by Ultrasound

JOHN THACKER

Changes in the inherited characteristics of living organisms occur naturally through an inability to maintain and reproduce their hereditary material (DNA) with absolute fidelity. Organisms also suffer natural or "spontaneous" damaging events from their environment which increase the probability of hereditary change. The frequency with which these changes occur in human populations is only known imprecisely, but it is generally accepted that most such changes, and any increase in their frequency, will be harmful.[1-3] Many physical and chemical agents in current production and use are known to cause hereditary changes; exposure to given levels of these agents may be found acceptable because the benefits of their use considerably outweigh their hereditary consequences. It is in this context that the medical use of ultrasound must be considered: it has evident benefits, but some (therapeutic) applications are effective because ultrasound can modify tissue responses. Does this suggest that ultrasound treatments may also lead to an increase in the frequency of hereditary changes? To answer this question meaningfully we must be aware of both the possible mechanisms by which ultrasound can cause damage to biological material and the nature of hereditary changes.

Classically, the term "mutation" is used to denote an inherited change in a cell or organism, and the nature of the change is established through breeding or lineage analysis. However, with the identification of the hereditary material at the microscopic (chromosome) and molecular (DNA) levels, a variety of changes observed directly in the hereditary material have been termed "genetic changes" or even "mutations." Some of these changes, such as chromosome or DNA breakage, may not be inherited (often because they are lethal) and others, such as certain types of chromosome recombinations, may not be of hereditary consequence to the cell or organism. These types of change may, however, be taken as indicators of possible damage leading to hereditary changes and as such have been used as the basis of a number of test systems introduced in the last few years.[4] The test systems allow simple and inexpensive checking of potential mutagenic agents, especially new chemicals, but care must be taken in the interpretation of results since the inference that nonhereditary damage to DNA or chromosomes indicates the potential for hereditary changes may not be true for all agents. As one illustration of this problem, studies on damage to DNA in solution by ultrasound will first be considered.

DAMAGE TO DNA IN SOLUTION EXPOSED TO ULTRASOUND

The observation that ultrasound can degrade DNA in solution has led to claims that it would be surprising if this "had no genetic consequences under some, if not all, conditions"[5] or, more directly, that "sonication is mutagenic for purified DNA."[6] However, a critical review of the experimental evidence on DNA degradation[7] shows that it is consistent with a mechanism involving hydrodynamic shear forces generated by cavitation phenomena. That is, ultrasound stimulates the oscillation of gas bubbles in aqueous solutions which in turn sets up velocity gradients into which DNA molecules may be drawn (see Chapter 3). DNA in solution is relatively free of constraints restricting its ability to respond to hydrodynamic forces: molecules will tend to extend linearly, become mechanically strained, and eventually shear at a point around their centers when the velocity gradient exceeds a certain threshold value. This damage to DNA can be shown to occur at relatively low intensity thresholds; for example, one detailed study[8] with continuous-wave (CW) ultrasound at a frequency of 1 MHz showed that degradation began at spatial-average intensities exceeding 400 mW/cm², when high-molecular-weight DNA was sonicated for 3 minutes under conditions stabilizing the cavitational field. Does this degradation have hereditary consequences, however? One direct test has been made (in vitro): Combes[9] exposed genetically marked DNA in solution to ultrasound and subsequently examined the DNA for mutation of the marker genes (using a technique whereby the DNA could be taken up into bacterial cells for marker gene expression). This technique is able to detect with considerable sensitivity the mutagenic activity of different chemical and physical agents, while showing a very low frequency of spontaneous mutations.[10] However, no mutations were found in very large numbers of bacteria expressing ultrasound-treated DNA (spatial peak intensities of 5 W/cm² and 10 W/cm² continuous-mode at 1 MHz for up to 20 minutes, or spatial-peak temporal-average intensity (SPTA intensity; see Chapter 2) 40 mW/cm² at 1.5 MHz in pulses of 20 μsec on:5 msec off for up to 20 minutes).[9]

In relating this mode of damage to cells and organisms it should be noted that DNA in vivo is intimately associated with proteins which determine a specific supercoiled configuration giving much less flexibility for mechanical disruption. The effective viscosity (shear modulus) of the cellular matrix is also greater than that of dilute aqueous solutions, so that the ultrasound intensity required to generate a given shear deformation will be correspondingly greater.[11] Thus at intensities likely to cause DNA damage of the type reported above, cells and organisms would suffer disruption of any mechanically-fragile structures (e.g., membranes). General cell and tissue disruption, rather than selective effects on DNA and chromosomes, might be predicted to result from this type of action.

DAMAGE TO ISOLATED CELLS EXPOSED TO ULTRASOUND

Effects on DNA inside cells may be studied, for example, by the use of highly-sensitive probes which recognize single-stranded regions (SSRs) in the DNA double helix.[12] Single-stranded regions occur commonly when cells are synthesizing DNA but are relatively infrequent in other phases of the cell cycle (some SSRs will always be present, associated with transcription, recombination, and repair of DNA). One technique suggested to detect SSRs—measuring binding of an antibody specific to certain nucleic acid bases—was employed by Liebeskind et al.[13] in vitro to show that ultrasound gave an increase in the frequency of antibody binding to non-DNA-synthesizing human cells (SPTA intensity 15 mW/cm^2 at 2.5 MHz in pulses of 3 μsec on: 5 msec off for 20 min). The ability to bind the antibody quickly returned to normal in ultrasound-treated cells but it was also possible to detect in some experiments a concomitant stimulation of DNA (repair ?) synthesis. The potential importance of these data is their indication that diagnostic levels of ultrasound might damage DNA to an extent stimulating cellular repair processes, which might in turn indicate a potential for hereditary changes. However, the interpretation of these experiments is complicated by lack of knowledge of the specificity of the antibody probe (it has not been shown under cellular conditions to bind only to single-strand DNA and will under some circumstances bind to RNA), by the inability to show in all experiments a concomitant stimulation of DNA synthesis, and by the finding that under the same conditions ultrasound did not induce DNA single-strand breaks measured by a sensitive centrifugation technique.[13] Additionally in an independent study with a different but more specific method for measuring SSRs in DNA—using an endonuclease enzyme which only cuts DNA at single-stranded sites, converting them to double-strand breaks which can be scored as chromosome damage—Wegner et al.[14] showed no increase after ultrasound treatment of mammalian cells (stated "output" 10 mW/cm^2 at 2.2 MHz). Although there were other methodological differences between these two studies (cell type, cell phase treated, mode of treatment), the latter result is perhaps more relevant to the question of hereditary damage in showing that SSRs leading to chromosomal changes are not induced by ultrasound.

From studies of microbial cells (yeast,[15] bacteria[16]) differing in their capacities to repair DNA damage, there has been no evidence of a correlation between DNA repair capacity and sensitivity to the lethal (cavitational) effects of ultrasound.

Two of the above groups of investigators[13, 14] have also studied the effect of ultrasound on a simple chromosome response, namely, sister chromatid exchange (SCE). How SCEs arise is not well understood, but their measurement is favoured as a test system for its ability to detect the DNA-damaging activity of many known mutagenic agents.[17] Sister chromatid exchange itself does not have any known hereditary consequences, and is poor for the detection of some mutagens such as x- or γ-rays (indeed, ionizing radiation alone may not be able to induce SCEs[18-20]). Liebeskind et al.[13] found no increase in the frequency of SCEs after ultrasound treatment of an established line of human cells (exposure parameters as above),[13] but subsequently observed a small but consistent increase in SCE frequency in ultrasound-treated human lymphocytes and lymphoblastoid cells (SPTA intensity up to 5 mW/cm² at 2 MHz for 30 minutes).[21] The increased frequency found was, on average, less than 1.5 times the spontaneous SCE frequency. However, using cultured hamster cells, which are similar to or more sensitive than human cells to SCE induction,[17] Wegner et al.[14] found no increase in SCE frequency after ultrasound treatment (exposure parameters as above). This negative report is supported by two other reports, one for human lymphocytes (spatial-peak intensities of 15–36 W/cm² at 1 MHz for 10 minutes)[22] and the other for hamster cells (SPTA intensities of 0.1–4.5 W/cm² at 3 MHz for 5 minutes or 30 minutes),[23] in which ultrasound treatment induced no significant increase in SCE frequency. All together, sufficient similarity in methods is found in these studies of SCE induction to suggest that differences in treatment or measurement conditions cannot explain the one positive result. (See Chapter 4 for further discussion of SCE induction.)

These findings are reminiscent of those from an earlier set of studies on "classical" chromosome aberration induction by ultrasound in human lymphocytes and other cultured mammalian cells. Thus in the early 1970s, Macintosh and Davey[24, 25] reported a substantial induction of chromosome aberrations in human lymphocytes exposed to an ultrasonic fetal heart detector, but this result was not upheld by a large number of subsequent studies. Independent reports from investigators employing a range of exposure parameters (pulsed and continuous modes with intensities used in both diagnosis and therapy at frequencies from 0.8–3 MHz) failed to detect an increase in aberration frequency.[26-35] A study of the chromosomes of newborn infants after fetal heart monitoring also showed no increase in the frequency of aberrations in lymphocytes.[36] In addition, a later study by Macintosh and others,[37] carefully reproducing the conditions of his original (positive) experiments, showed no increase in aberration frequency; these investigators concluded that an unidentified artefact was responsible for aberration induction in the original experiments.

The studies summarized above highlight the need for considerable care in the interpretation of reports of ultrasound-induced bioeffects; to interpret reliably such data a thorough understanding of the measured response is required. Failing this, there must be a substantial consensus of experimental data from independent investigators using rigorously applied methods to support a positive effect in a system known to detect other mutagenic agents. In these terms, none of the above positive reports can be considered to indicate a potential genetic hazard from diagnostic levels of ultrasound. This conclusion is supported by studies on the induction of mutations in cells, which will be considered next.

The measurement of mutations in microbes can now be made with relative ease, and the basic methods have in the last few years been successfully applied to isolated mammalian cells. However, the suitability of available cell mutation systems for testing ultrasound varies; in some systems mutation is only detectable if a specific type of small DNA base alteration is induced by the agent being tested. Experiments on the effect of ultrasound on bacterial cell mutation mostly fall into this category. Thus, Combes[9] studied mutation to tryptophan-independence in the bacterium *Bacillus subtilis;* this mutation requires a specific intragenic change (or possibly a second-site suppressor) and occurs at a spontaneous frequency of about $1/10^8$ cells examined. No significant increase in mutation frequency was detected among cells treated with ultrasound (SPTA intensities of 40–240 mW/cm² at 2 MHz in 20 μsec on:5 msec off periods for up to 20 minutes). Barnett et al.[23] exposed five *Salmonella typhimurium* bacterial test strains to ultrasound; some of these strains require specific DNA base substitutions while others require DNA base deletion or addition before a mutation is detected. Again no significant increase in mutant numbers was found for any of these strains after ultrasound treatment (SPTA intensities of 0.1–4.5 W/cm² at 3 MHz for 5 minutes or 30 minutes); although mutant frequency (mutants per viable cell) was not monitored accurately it was unlikely to have been altered by these exposure conditions. In a more extensive study using the eukaryotic microbe *Saccharomyces cerevisiae* (yeast), which has a cellular structure more closely resembling higher cell types than bacteria, Thacker[15] measured mutation and recombination frequencies after ultrasound treatment (spatial-peak temporal-average intensities of 40 mW/cm² or 600 mW/cm² at 1–2 MHz with 20 μsec on:5 msec off periods for 5–20 or 120 minutes, respectively; and continuous-mode 3–5 W/cm² at 1 MHz for up to 30 minutes). The mutations measured in this study embraced a wider range of potential DNA alterations, and included mutation of both nuclear and mitochondrial DNA, as well as mitotic recombination (change in the distribution of hereditary material which can under some circumstances lead to the exposure of previously concealed genes having deleterious effects). The frequency of all these hereditary effects was not found to be increased by ultrasound, even under treatment conditions where cavitation phenomena were generated and cells killed. Only where long exposures to CW ultrasound at high intensities generated sufficient heat or free radicals (and hydrogen peroxide) was there an increase in the frequency of some types of mutation.[15] Similarly, Kaufman[38] has briefly reported that hamster cells exposed to 1-MHz CW ultrasound show no increase in mutant frequency at a spatial-peak intensity of 7 W/cm² but show a small frequency increase at 35 W/cm². He attributed this induction to free radicals formed by cavitational phenomena.

Finally a note should be made of an attempt to induce mammalian cell transformation by ultrasound (SPTA intensity 15 mW/cm² at 2.5 MHz for 20–40 minutes).[13] Cell transformation is considered to be one of the steps involved in the formation of tumors in vivo, and it was found that the frequency of morphologically transformed cells was increased by ultrasound in several experiments. Judgment on this result must be reserved at present, however, because it has been shown recently that the formation of transformed cell foci in density-inhibited cultures is subject to cell density effects which seriously discredit any quantitative measurements with current methods.[39]

DAMAGE TO DNA IN SOLUTION EXPOSED TO ULTRASOUND

In plant tissue exposed to ultrasound, damage to chromosomes has been reported at intensities above 1 W/cm² continuous-mode at 1–2 MHz.[7] Work in the 1950s suggested that this damage is due to intratissue cavitation or, at some intensities, heating effects which rapidly lead to cell death and leave surviving cells with no chromosome abnormalities. Recent studies have supported this conclusion: none of the "classical" forms of chromosome aberration, induced by such agents as ionizing radiation and various chemical mutagens, were observed after ultrasound exposure.[40, 41] The types of damage described[40-42]—"bridging" and clumping of chromosomes—are not generally associated with inherited changes. Plant tissue seems to be especially vulnerable to the cavitational effects of ultrasound because of the presence of gas-filled spaces between cells.[43, 44] Few reports of similar damage to mammalian tissue have been made, but Woeber[45] noted chromosome disruption and clumping in rat carcinoma tissue treated with 0.5–4.5 W/cm² at 1 MHz for 3–5 minutes.

The effects of ultrasound on mutation frequency in multicellular organisms have been investigated in the fruit fly (*Drosophila*) and in mice. *Drosophila melanogaster* has been extensively characterized and developed for mutation studies over many years. Two studies with ultrasound in recent years may be cited: Fritz-Niggli and Böni[46] examined the progeny of treated eggs, larvae, and pupae for sex-linked lethal mutations but found little or no induction at intensities of 0.3–1.75 W/cm² continuous-mode at 0.8 MHz for up to 25 minutes (insufficient numbers were examined to establish the spontaneous frequency). More recently, Thacker and Baker[47] treated adult flies of this species with spatial-peak intensities of 50 mW/cm² continuous-mode for 60 min or 0.5–2 W/cm² continuous-mode for 2–10 minutes (1 MHz) and measured recessive lethal mutations and nondisjunction in large-scale breeding experiments with flies surviving treatment. Nondisjunction is a consequence of disturbance in the regular pattern of separation of chromosomes at cell division, and can lead to loss or gain of whole chromosomes (*aneuploidy*). Aneuploidy is associated with as much as one-quarter of human spontaneous abortions and about 0.4 percent of live births.[48] Recessive lethal mutations could be caused by a variety of DNA alterations, from small base changes within genes to deletions or rearrangements of whole genes, but no increase in the frequency of these mutations or of nondisjunction was found after ultrasound treatment.[47] Heat rise within the flies was only 1–2°C at the highest intensity used in this study.

Lyon and Simpson[49] carried out extensive tests for damage in the gonads of male and female mice exposed to 1.5-MHz ultrasound for 15 minutes. Intensities were either spatial-average 1.6 W/cm² continuous-mode, or spatial-average temporal-average 1.6 W/cm² in pulses of 1 msec on:3 msec off (males only), or spatial-average temporal-average 0.9 W/cm² in pulses of 30 μsec on:1 msec off. Temperature rises of 1–2°C were recorded at the skin surface. In males, no reduction in testis weight or sperm count, no induction of chromosome aberrations in spermatocytes, and no increase in the frequency of dominant lethal mutations (measured as postimplantation loss of embryos from matings with treated males) or sterility was found for up to 8 weeks after exposure. A large variation in the preimplantation survival was found among embryos sired by males exposed to the 30-μsec pulses, but the controls showed similar variation at different times and it was considered that failures in fertilization were responsible. Similarly, in females exposed several days before mating and up to the time of mating, there was no increase in the dominant lethal mutation frequency, although a significant increase in the frequency of sterile matings was found for continuous-mode treatment on the day of mating and for treatments with 30-μsec pulses on 1 to several days prior to mating. These results gave no indication of any genetic damage to mice gonads from the ultrasound treatments, while parallel x-ray treatments gave characteristic (if small) increases in all the tests.

CONCLUSION

Overall the data reviewed above provide little evidence that ultrasound treatment will lead to an increased frequency of inherited changes. This is not to say that the tests for inherited changes are complete—indeed, part of the purpose of this review is to make the concerned reader aware that new tests are continually being devised and some of these will undoubtedly be used to assess possible risks from ultrasound treatment. As emphasized above, some knowledge of the way in which ultrasound can cause biological effects and of the biological basis of the test system are required if meaningful estimates of risk are to be derived. At present there are no valid means of testing for potential mutagenic activity in the tissue of ultimate concern, the human gonads; thus, in common with studies of other potential mutagenic agents, there is a further problem of extrapolation of data from the available test systems to effects in man.[50] It is difficult, however, to envisage a mechanism of damage by ultrasound which will operate exclusively in human tissue.

In terms of clinical practice, the few definite reports of damage to the genetic material occur at intensities and/or durations of treatment that are well in excess of those used in diagnostic applications. Secondary phenomena, such as cavitation or heating, have usually been implicated in the production of this damage. The likelihood that cavitational effects will be generated in mammalian tissue is still in dispute, although it is argued above that mechanical forces associated with cavitation will not act selectively on DNA and chromosomes and will most probably lead to cell death rather than inherited changes. However, cavitation may also generate some free radicals and peroxides which can have weak mutagenic effects. Additionally, and probably more importantly, significant heat rise will occur in tissue with prolonged treatment at high intensities, and heat shock can also have mutagenic effects.[7]

On this basis, the argument for a lack of risk from diagnostic applications may appear to rest upon the assumption that there are intensity and/or time thresholds for the induction of hereditary changes. Certainly such thresholds seem to exist for the induction by ultrasound of certain sensitive responses in mammalian tissue (e.g., see Dunn and Fry[51]), and it is possible that these reflect thresholds for the production of secondary phenomena such as cavitation or heating. However, even if thresholds did not exist, it seems very unlikely on present evidence that current diagnostic applications will lead to frequencies of inherited changes that will exceed their natural frequency in man.

REFERENCES

1. Edwards JH: The cost of mutation. p. 465. In Berg K (ed): Genetic Damage in Man Caused by Environmental Agents. Academic Press, New York, 1979

2. Childs JD: The effect of a change in mutation rate on the incidence of dominant and X-linked recessive disorders in man. Mutat Res 83:145, 1981

3. Neel JV: Frequency of spontaneous and induced 'point' mutations in higher eukaryotes. J Hered 74:2, 1983

4. Hollstein M, McCann J, Angelosanto FA, Nichols WW: Short term tests for carcinogens and mutagens. Mutat Res 65:133, 1979

5. Peacocke AR, Pritchard NJ: Some biophysical aspects of ultrasound. Prog Biophys Mol Biol 18:187, 1968

6. Galperin-Lemaitre H, Kirsch-Volders M, Levi S: Ultrasound and mammalian DNA. Lancet 2:662, 1975

7. Thacker J: The possibility of genetic hazard from ultrasonic radiation. Curr Topics Radiat Res Q 8:235, 1973

8. Hill CR, Clarke PR, Crowe MR, Hammick JW: Biophysical effects of cavitation in a 1 MHZ ultrasonic beam. p. 26. In Ultrasonics for Industry Conference Papers. Illife, London, 1969

9. Combes RD: Absence of mutation following ultrasonic treatment of Bacillus subtilis cells and transforming DNA. Br J Radiol 48:306, 1975

10. Bresler SE, Kalanin VL, Perumov DA: Inactivation and mutation of isolated DNA. II. Kinetics of mutagenesis and efficiency of various mutagens. Mutat Res 5:1, 1968

11. Hill CR: Ultrasonic exposure thresholds for changes in cells and tissues. J Acoust Soc Am 52:667, 1972

12. Wells RD, Goodman TC, Hillen W, et al: DNA structure and gene regulation. Prog Nucl Acids Res 24:167, 1980

13. Liebeskind D, Bases R, Elequin F, et al: Diagnostic ultrasound: effects on the DNA and growth patterns of animal cells. Radiology 131:177, 1979

14. Wegner RD, Obe G, Meyenburg M: Has diagnostic ultrasound mutagenic effects? Hum Genet 56:95, 1980

15. Thacker J: An assessment of ultrasonic radiation hazard using yeast genetic systems. Br J Radiol 47:130, 1974

16. Hedges M, Lewis M, Lunec J, Cramp WA: The effect of ultrasound at 1.5 MHz on *Escherichia coli*. Int J Radiat Biol 37:103, 1980

17. Perry PE: Chemical mutagens and sister chromatid exchange. p. 1. In de Serres FJ, Hollaender

A (eds): Chemical Mutagens. Principles and Methods for Their Detection. Vol. 6. Plenum Press, New York, 1980

18. Littlefield LG, Colyer SP, Joiner EE, DuFrain RJ: Sister chromatid exchanges in human lymphocytes exposed to ionising radiation during G_0. Radiat Res 78:514, 1979

19. Barjaktarović N, Savage JRK: RBE for d(42 MeV)-Be neutrons based on chromosome-type aberrations induced in human lymphocytes and scored in cells at first division. Int J Radiat Biol 37:667, 1980

20. Duncan AMV, Evans HJ: Gamma irradiation of human peripheral lymphocytes: effects of low and prolonged irradiation on sister chromatid exchange induction. Int J Radiat Biol 43:175, 1983

21. Liebeskind D, Bases R, Mendez F, et al: Sister chromatid exchanges in human lymphocytes after exposure to diagnostic ultrasound. Science 205:1273, 1979

22. Morris SM, Palmer CG, Fry FJ, Johnson LK: Effect of ultrasound on human leucocytes. Sister chromatid exchange analysis. Ultrasound Med Biol 4:253, 1978

23. Barnett SB, Bonin A, Mitchell G, et al: An investigation of the mutagenic potential of pulsed ultrasound. Br J Radiol 55:501, 1982

24. Macintosh IJC, Davey DA: Chromosome aberrations induced by an ultrasonic fetal pulse detector. Br Med J 4:92, 1970

25. Macintosh IJC, Davey DA: Relationship between intensity of ultrasound and induction of chromosome aberrations. Br J Radiol 45:320, 1972

26. Boyd E, Abdulla U, Donald I, et al: Chromosome breakage and ultrasound. Br Med J 2:501, 1971

27. Bobrow M, Blackwell N, Unrau AE, Bleaney B: Absence of any observed effect of ultrasonic irradiation on human chromosomes. J Obstet Gynecol 78:730, 1971

28. Buckton KE, Baker NV: An investigation into possible chromosome damaging effects of ultrasound on human blood cells. Br J Radiol 45:340, 1972

29. Coakley WT, Slade JS, Braeman JM, Moore JL: Examination of lymphocytes for chromosome aberrations after ultrasonic irradiation. Br J Radiol 45:328, 1972

30. Hill CR, Joshi GP, Revell SH: A search for chromosome damage following exposure of Chinese hamster cells to high intensity pulsed ultrasound. Br J Radiol 45:333, 1972

31. Watts PL, Hall AJ, Fleming JEE: Ultrasound and chromosome damage. Br J Radiol 45:335, 1972

32. Abdulla U, Talbert D, Lucas M, Mullarkey M: Effect of ultrasound on chromosomes of lymphocyte cultures. Br Med J 3:797, 1972

33. Galperin-Lemaitre H, Gustot P, Levi S: Ultrasound and marrow-cell chromosomes. Lancet 2:505, 1973

34. Brock RD, Peacock WJ, Geard CR, et al: Ultrasound and chromosome aberrations. Med J Austr 2:533, 1973

35. Rott HD, Soldner R: The effect of ultrasound on human chromosomes in vitro. Humangenetik 25:103, 1973

36. Lucas M, Mullarkey M, Abdulla U: Study of chromosomes in the newborn after ultrasonic fetal heart monitoring in labour. Br Med J 3:795, 1972

37. Macintosh IJC, Brown RC, Coakley WT: Ultrasound and in vitro chromosome aberrations. Br J Radiol 48:230, 1975

38. Kaufman GE: Ultrasound is a weak mutagen in mammalian cells. Radiat Res 91:368, 1982

39. Kennedy AR, Fox M, Murphy G, Little JB: Relationship between X-ray exposure and malignant transformation in C3H 10T½ cells. Proc Natl Acad Sci USA 77:7262, 1980

40. Gregory WD, Miller MW, Carstensen EL, et al: Nonthermal effects of 2 MHz ultrasound on the growth and cytology of Vicia faba roots. Br J Radiol 47:122, 1974

41. Khokhar MT, Oliver R: An investigation of chromosome damage in *Vicia faba* root tips after exposure to 1.5 MHz ultrasonic radiation. Int J Radiat Biol 28:373, 1975

42. Cataldo FL, Miller MW, Gregory WD, Carstensen EL: A description of ultrasonically-induced chromosome anomalies in *Vicia faba*. Radiat Bot 13:211, 1973

43. Gershoy A, Miller DL, Nyborg WL: Intercellular gas: its role in sonated plant tissue. p. 501. In White D, Barnes R (eds): Ultrasound in Medicine. Vol 2. Plenum Press, New York, 1976

44. Miller DL: The botanical effects of ultrasound: a review. Environ Exp Bot 23:1, 1983

45. Woeber K: Histologische untersuchungen über die Sofortreaktion des Zellkerns beim Walkerkarzinom der Ratte nach Ultraschalleinwirkung. Strahlentherapie 85:207, 1951

46. Fritz-Niggli H, Böni A: Biological experiments on *Drosophila melanogaster* with supersonic vibrations. Science 112:120, 1950

47. Thacker J, Baker NV: The use of *Drosophila* to estimate the possibility of genetic hazard from ultrasound irradiations. Br J Radiol 49:367, 1976

48. Nielsen J, Sillesen I: Incidence of chromosome aberrations among 11,148 newborn children. Hum Genet 30:1, 1975

49. Lyon MF, Simpson GM: An investigation into the possible genetic hazards of ultrasound. Br J Radiol 47:712, 1974

50. Streisinger G: Extrapolations from species to species and from various cell types in assessing risks from chemical mutagens. Mutat Res 114:93, 1983

51. Dunn F, Fry FJ: Ultrasonic threshold dosages for the mammalian central nervous system. IEEE Trans Biomed Eng 18:253, 1971

7 Biological Effects in Laboratory Animals

WILLIAM D. O'BRIEN, JR.

In animal studies, attention has been given to a number of ultrasonically induced biological effect end-points. One can think of these as being classified into one of two general categories: structural or functional alterations. A change in biological material that is determined through histologic means is considered a morphologic or structural alteration. Most ultrasonically induced structural alterations have been assessed by light microscopy. A biological effect which is assessed by a change in some biochemical level, pH, or activity is considered a functional alteration. In general, relatively high ultrasonic intensity levels are required to produce a structural alteration; at lower levels, where structural alterations are not detectable, functional alterations have been observed.

In the context of a structural or functional alteration, there are various degrees to which the experimental data are conflicting. One category of observations deals mainly with structural alterations (usually termed "lesions" here) of biological tissues produced by quite high levels of ultrasonic energy. Here there is no conflict in terms of whether or not a specific effect occurred but there are conflicting viewpoints in terms of the fundamental mechanism or mechanisms responsible. At lower ultrasonic energy levels, usually within the therapeutic range, there are conflicting viewpoints as to whether, or to what degree, a structural alteration occurred. And, for a third general category, at ultrasonic energy levels lower than the therapeutic range, sometimes at diagnostic levels, there are no indications of structural changes and there are very conflicting data as to whether a functional alteration occurred.

HIGH-INTENSITY ULTRASONIC STUDIES

Some 35 years after the Curies discovered piezoelectricity in 1880,[1] the French scientist Paul Langevin developed the first use of ultrasonic energy wherein underwater acoustic echoes were bounced off of submerged objects.[2,3] During the course of this work, the first reported observation was made that ultrasonic energy had a lethal effect upon small aquatic animals.[4] The first extensive investigation of the phenomena observed by Langevin was conducted by Wood and Loomis.[5] Although the ultrasonic levels were not specified, they did confirm Langevin's observation that ultrasonic energy could kill small fishes and frogs by exposures of 1–2 minutes. In perhaps the first review study, Harvey (1930)[6] examined physical, chemical, and biological effects of ultrasound; effects on cells, isolated cells, bacteria, and tissues were summarized with a view toward identifying the responsible mechanism. The ultrasonic exposure conditions of this early work were not well characterized or reported at all but the intensity levels were undoubtedly quite high.

A gap of almost two decades existed before ultrasonic biophysical studies began to provide an insight into the mechanisms by which ultrasonic energy altered biological materials. Generally, the ultrasonic intensity levels employed in these studies to elicit a well-defined and reproducible biological effect were quite high.

The early pioneering studies of W. J. Fry and colleagues,[7, 8] in which the ultrasonic exposure conditions were carefully controlled and specified, examined the production and mechanisms of sciatic nerve paralysis in the frog. In most cases, these studies represented rather gross damage because the ultrasonic energy induced immediate structural alterations. Later Fry[9] reviewed the production of ultrasonically induced lesions in central nervous system tissue using focused ultrasonic energy. These studies provided important basic information which led to additional studies of the effects of intense ultrasound upon the mammalian central nervous system.[10-15] Fundamental findings in terms of *dosimetry* (quantitative assessment of the ultrasonic exposure required to elicit a specific biological effect) and in terms of *mechanisms* (causes for biological effects) resulted from these animal studies.

Studies at high intensities present some limitations for assessing potential effects, or lack of them, at ultrasonic levels employed in clinical medicine. However, these studies support the view that the ultrasonic exposure conditions employed diagnostically more than likely will not produce acute, gross irreversible damage to the irradiated tissue.

At present, high-intensity studies are continuing in order to understand the bases for structural alterations at the electron microscope level.[16, 17] It appears that the ultrasonic levels necessary to produce a detectable structural alteration are less when assessed with electron microscopy as compared with light microscopy.

LOWER-INTENSITY ULTRASONIC STUDIES

At somewhat lower ultrasonic levels than those employed above, structural alterations to ovarian and testicular tissue have been studied in experimental animals. Morphologic alteration of cells was observed in mouse ovaries exposed to ultrasonic spatial-peak temporal-average (SPTA—see Chapter 2) intensities of 25 W/cm² and above when the ovaries were examined at least 24 hours after ultrasonic exposure; no lesions were detected in animals killed immediately after the ovaries were exposed to ultrasound. Lesions were also absent from ovaries exposed to SPTA intensities of 5–10 W/cm² but abnormalities here suggested the occurrence of more subtle types of alteration. It was observed that the morphologic alterations due to ultrasound were very similar to those of ionizing radiation, the difference being in the sensitivity of the various ovarian elements to the insult. These findings suggested that luteinized cells were preferentially damaged by ultrasound, by contrast to the effect of ionizing radiation.[18]

Conflicting reports have appeared from animal studies wherein ultrasound has been found in some studies to affect spermatogenesis and fertility[19, 20] and where in other studies no such effects were observed.[21] Thus, the few data available for basing an assessment of risk to testicular tissue from ultrasonic energy are contradictory.

It has been shown[22] that in vivo ultrasonically (1 MHz) irradiated mouse testes, exposed for 30 seconds at a spatial-peak intensity of 25 W/cm² exhibited two types of damage, namely, seminiferous tubule damage, with a suggestion of minor intertubule space involvement, and a more severe form of tubule damage, with significant interstitial involvement. The damage at the cellular level varied, depending upon the types of cell examined. In the case of ionizing radiation, the order of sensitivity of germ cells is known,[23, 24] and at least initially, it is different for damage caused by ultrasound. Observations of the damage produced by ultrasound shows spermatocytes to be the first affected of any cell types in the testes.

A further study[25] was undertaken with a view toward identification of more subtle and/or alternate forms of testicular morphologic changes, at the lower spatial-peak intensities of 2 W/cm² and 5 W/cm², as well as classification of types of intratubular damage resulting from ultrasonic exposure. Morphologic alterations due to exposure to ultrasound at the low intensities appear to differ in some respects from effects of higher intensities.[22] First, no gradation of tubular involvement was seen, but altered tubules were randomly scattered throughout the sections and no visible estimate could be made of which side of the testis was facing the source of ultrasound. Second, the lacework appearance of tubules and gapping between cells reported at 25 W/cm² was rarely seen at the lower intensities of 5 W/cm² and 2 W/cm². Finally, periodic-acid Schiff (PAS)-positive materials, acrosomes in particular, were present and normal in all but heavily damaged tubules, which suggests a continuance of spermiogenesis not seen at higher intensities[22] or at much longer exposure times.[26] Observed differences in extent and in type of alterations between the two intensities of exposure used were considered not significant.

FETAL STUDIES—HIGH AND LOW ULTRASONIC INTENSITIES

The early studies dealing with the effects of ultrasound on fetal growth and development and on fetal abnormalities were quite conflicting. High-level ultrasonic exposures of pregnant mice yielded negative findings whereas reports of pregnant mice and rats ultrasonically exposed at lower levels, diagnostic levels in some cases, suggested the possibility of structural and/or functional alterations of the fetuses.

In one series of experiments,[27, 28] pregnant mice were exposed to pulsed ultrasound under a wide variety of exposure conditions where the maximum intensity (I_m—see Chapter 2) ranged from 20 to 490 W/cm^2, the spatial-peak temporal-average (SPTA) intensity ranged from 0.75 to 27 W/cm^2, and the exposure time was typically 300 seconds. The investigators concluded that there was no significant effect on litter size, resorption rate, or abnormality rate.

In what was perhaps one of the more controversial studies of its time, Shoji et al.[29, 30] investigated the effects of prenatal ultrasonic exposure of pregnant mice. Pregnant DHS mice were irradiated on the ninth day of gestation with continuous-wave (CW) (2.25 MHz) ultrasound for a period of 5 hours at a reported intensity (presumably spatial average) of 40 mW/cm^2. The signal source was a commercial fetal Doppler device and no dosimetric details were provided. Eight types of fetal abnormalities were observed in both the irradiated and control groups, with no significant differences in the rates of their occurrence between the two groups. However, the rate of fetal death was significantly higher in the irradiated group.[29] Later, Shoji et al. reported a statistically significant increase in fetal abnormalities in a different mouse strain, A/He, and reported a significant effect of fetal mortality.[30, 31] In both of these studies, mice were given an initial dose of sodium nembutal which was effective for approximately 1 hour, after which the animals struggled. Lele[32] suggested that these observations were consistent with results of prolonged induction of a moderate temperature rise. Nyborg[33] observed that Lele's temperature measurements were similar to those predicted by a theoretical plot of temperature at the center of an absorbing sphere.

Mannor[34] examined the effect of in utero CW (2.28 MHz) ultrasonic irradiation of pregnant mice during gestational ages from 8 to 16 days at spatial-average intensities of 0.16, 0.27, 0.49, and 1.05 W/cm^2 and exposure times of 5 and 10 minutes. Some maternal deaths were attributed to heat at the higher exposure conditions. All fetuses examined in surviving females were reported to be normal. McClain et al.[35] studied the effects of multiple prenatal exposure from a commercial prototype of a fetal Doppler device (CW, 2.5 MHz, spatial-average intensity of 9.1 mW/cm^2 in rats). Examination of the fetuses on the 20th day of gestation showed no significant differences in fetal and maternal weight, viability, death, litter size, implants, and external and soft tissue abnormalities.

One of the more comprehensive investigations of fetal weight reduction in mice ultrasonically exposed in utero has resulted in a dose-effect observation which can be applied to making an assessment of risk relative to this functional alteration. The earliest of the studies[36] suggested that in utero ultrasonic irradiation affected prenatal growth and development. Time-mated CF$_1$ mice were irradiated to CW (1 MHz) ultrasound on the eighth day of gestation. The fetuses were removed by laparotomy on the 18th day of gestation and individually weighed. The data showed a statistically significant fetal weight reduction from about 6 to 18 percent, depending upon the exposure conditions. There were seven exposure groups, including a sham. Two hundred and seventy-two litters (2,866 fetuses) were exposed under conditions ranging from 0.5 to 5.5 W/cm² for the spatially averaged intensity (I) and from 10 to 300 seconds for the exposure time (t). A dose-effect dependence of exposure condition versus average fetal weight was examined by defining the dose parameter I^2t.[37]

The observation that in utero ultrasonic exposure of mice can cause weight reduction in fetuses compared with the sham has also been confirmed by two other groups using two different strains of mice, namely, LAF_1/J mice[38,39] and CFW Swiss-Webster mice.[40] In the earlier study,[38] relatively high-level pulsed ultrasound conditions (center frequency around 1 MHz) were employed, and a significant reduction in fetal weight was reported for SPTA intensities above 50 W/cm² [maximum intensity (I_m) of 2,936 W/cm²] and exposure times of 20 seconds when fetuses were irradiated on the eighth day of gestation. The later report by Fry et al.[39] indicated that the highest exposure conditions [maximum intensity (I_m) of 1,936 W/cm², SPTA intensity of 51 W/cm², and exposure time of 20 seconds] produced a statistically significant 18.8 percent fetal weight reduction (relative to the sham animals), whereas at a SPTA intensity of 45 W/cm² and lower [maximum intensity (I_m) of 1,936 W/cm² and exposure time of 20 seconds], there was no change in the fetal weight relative to the sham. Stolzenberg et al.[40] reported on fetal weight reductions ranging up to 25 percent relative to the sham animals when the mice were ultrasonically exposed (CW 2 MHz, spatial-average intensity of 1 W/cm², exposure times up to 200 seconds) at gestational ages of 0, 7, or 12 days and examined on the 17th day of gestation.

A preliminary study conducted at even lower ultrasonic levels suggested that the fetal weight reduction may be sustained postweaning.[41] Time-mated CF_1 mice were irradiated at the 13th day of gestation with CW (1 MHz) ultrasound and examined at 55 days postconception (approximately 2 weeks postweaning). There were three exposure groups (sham, 0.25 W/cm², and 0.80 W/cm² spatial-average intensity, each for 120 seconds) and the data yielded statistically significant weight reductions of 8.7 percent and 14.8 percent, respectively, relatively to the sham. However, in a follow-up study, Stratmeyer et al.[42] did not confirm this earlier finding of sustained postweaning weight reduction. Rather, a weight gain compared to the sham was suggested. Fetal weight reduction was not observed in rats exposed on the ninth day of gestation to CW (3.2 MHz) ultrasound, even at exposure conditions that produced some mortality.[43] There were, however, a few pups stunted but this observation was not statistically significant.

For further discussion of fetal studies, see Chapters 8, 9, and 10.

CONCLUDING COMMENTS

An important concern deals with the question of the significance of an ultrasonically induced biological alteration, for example, as viewed with respect to risk. But very little effort has gone into the assessment of specific biological alterations. This is true, in part, because appropriate dose-effect responses of these alterations have not been developed. Rather, a single dosimetric condition has been utilized for the experiment and this has precluded our ability to investigate the role of that particular biological alteration in terms of extrapolating it from the experimental animal to human beings. Herein lies the greatest importance of investigating ultrasonically induced biological alterations in experimental animals. Such biological observations can provide insight into the risk, if any, to which humans might be subjected. Dose-effect observations provide the fundamental basis from which mechanisms of interaction can be determined and thus provide a firmer scientific basis for extrapolation to humans.

In conclusion, based upon experimental animal studies, it appears that the available information suggests that the risk associated with the clinical use of ultrasound is quite low. However, our knowledge regarding ultrasonic bioeffects and biophysical interaction is rather incomplete at this time. Because of this apparent paradox, it is essential for the clinicians to be provided with up-to-date information on potential risks so that they can continue to render an informed benefit-risk judgment. The principal source of such data is from animal experiments. It is difficult to evaluate any of these studies in isolation, especially when there are conflicting observations. And there will be conflicting observations especially as the ultrasonic levels decrease. This is a given and it must be understood.

ACKNOWLEDGMENTS

The work of the author described in this chapter was supported in part by a grant from the National Institutes of Health, National Institute of General Medical Sciences (GM 30481).

REFERENCES

1. Cady WG: Piezoelectricity. Vol. 1. Dover, New York, 1946
2. Urich RJ: Principles of Underwater Sound for Engineers. McGraw-Hill, New York, 1967
3. Van Went JM: Ultrasonic and Ultrashort Waves in Medicine. Elsevier, New York, 1954
4. Graber P: Biological actions of ultrasonic wave. p. 191. In Lawrence JH, Tobias CA (eds): Advances in Biological Physics. Vol. 3. Academic Press, New York, 1953
5. Wood RW, Loomis AL: The physical and biological effects of high-frequency sound-waves of great intensity. Phil Mag 4:417, 1927
6. Harvey EN: Biological aspects of ultrasonic waves, a general survey. Biol Bull 59:306, 1930
7. Fry WJ, Wulff VJ, Tucker D, et al: Physical factors involved in ultrasonically induced changes in living system: I. Identification of non-temperature effects. J Acoust Soc Am 22:867, 1950
8. Fry WJ, Tucker D, Fry FJ, et al: Physical factors involved in ultrasonically induced changes in living system: II. Amplitude duration relations and the effect of hydrostatic pressure for nerve tissue. J Acoust Soc Am 23:364, 1951
9. Fry WJ: Intense ultrasound in investigations of the central nervous system. Adv Biol Med Phys 6:281, 1958
10. Hueter TF, Ballantine HT, Jr, Cotter WC: Production of lesions in the central nervous system with focused ultrasound. A study of dosage factors. J Acoust Soc Am 28:192, 1956

11. Dunn F: Physical mechanisms of the action of intense ultrasound on tissue. Am J Phys Med 37:14, 1958

12. Fry FJ, Kosoff G, Eggleton RC, Dunn F: Threshold ultrasonic dosages for structural changes in the mammalian brain. J Acoust Soc Am 48:1413, 1970

13. Pond JB: The role of heat in the production of ultrasonic focal lesions, J Acoust Soc Am 47:1607, 1970

14. Dunn F, Fry FJ: Ultrasonic threshold dosages for the mammalian central nervous system. IEEE Trans Biomed Engl BME-18:253, 1971

15. Robinson TC, Lele PP: An analysis of lesion development in the brain and in plastics by high-intensity focused ultrasound at low-megahertz frequencies. J Acoust Soc Am 51:1333, 1972

16. Borrelli MJ, Bailey KI, Dunn F: Early ultrasonic effects upon mammalian CNS structures (chemical synapses). J Acoust Soc Am 69:1514, 1981

17. Frizzell LA, Lee CS, Aschenbach PD, et al: Involvement of ultrasonically induced cavitation in hind limb paralysis of the mouse neonate. J Acoust Soc Am 74:1062, 1983

18. Bailey KI, O'Brien WD, Dunn F: Ultrasonically induced morphological damage to mouse ovaries. Ultrasound Med Biol 9:25, 1983

19. Kamocsay D, Rona G, Tarnoczy T: Effects of ultrasonics on the testicles, experimental studies on white rats. Arzt Forch 9:389, 1955

20. Fahim MS, Fahim Z, Der R, et al: Heat in male contraception (hot water 60°C, infrared, microwave, and ultrasound. Contraception 11:549, 1975

21. Lyon MF, Simpson GM: An investigation into the possible genetic hazards of ultrasound. Br J Radiol 47:712, 1974

22. O'Brien WD, Brady JK, Dunn F: Morphological changes to mouse testicular tissue from in vivo ultrasonic irradiation. Ultrasound Med Biol 5:35, 1979

23. Oakberg EF: Duration of spermatogenesis in the mouse and timing of stages of the cycle of the seminiferous epithelium. Am J Anat 99:507, 1956

24. Mandl AM: The radio sensitivity of germ cells. Biol Rev 39:288, 1964

25. Bailey KI, O'Brien WD, Dunn F: Ultrasonically induced, in vivo morphological damage in mouse testicular tissue. Arch Androl 6:301, 1981

26. Dumontier A, Bierdick A, Ewigman B, Fahim MS: Effects of sonication on mature rat teste. Fertil Steril 28:196, 1977

27. Woodward B, Pond MB, Warwick R: How safe is diagnostic sonar. Br J Radiol 43:719, 1970

28. Warwick R, Pond JB, Woodward B, Connolly CC: Hazards of diagnostic ultrasonography— a study with mice. IEEE Trans Sonics Ultrasonics SU-17:158, 1970

29. Shoji R, Momma RE, Shimizu T, Matsuda S: An experimental study on the effect of low-intensity ultrasound on developing mouse embryos. J Fac Sci Hokkaido U Ser VI Zool 18:51, 1971

30. Shoji R, Momma T, Shimizu T, Matsuda S: Experimental studies on the effect of ultrasound on mouse embryos. Teratology 6:119, 1972

31. Shimizu T, Shoji R: Experimental safety study on mice exposed to low-intensity ultrasound. Presented at the 2nd Congress on Ultrasonics in Medicine, June 4–8, Rotterdam, The Netherlands, 1973

32. Lele PP: Ultrasonic teratology in mouse and man. p. 22. In: Ultrasonics in Medicine. Excerpta Medica Int Cong Series No. 363, Amsterdam, 1975

33. Nyborg WL: Physical mechanisms for biological effects of ultrasound. p. 84. In Repacholi MH, Benwell DA (eds): Ultrasound Short Course Transactions. Radiation Protection Bureau, Health Protection Branch, National Health and Welfare, Ottawa, Canada, 1979

34. Mannor SM, Serr DM, Ramari I, et al: The safety of ultrasound in fetal monitoring. Am J Obstet Gynecol 113:653, 1972

35. McClain RM, Hoar RM, Saltzman MB: Teratologic study of rats exposed to ultrasound. Am J Obstet Gynecol 114:39, 1972

36. O'Brien WD Jr: Ultrasonically induced fetal weight reduction in mice. P. 531. In White D, Barnes R (eds): Ultrasound in Medicine, Vol. 2. Plenum Press, New York, 1976

37. O'Brien WD, Jr: Dose-dependent effect of ultrasound on fetal weight of mice. J Ultrasound Med 2:1, 1983

38. Fry FJ, Johnson LK, Erdmann WA, et al: Ultrasonic toxicity in the mouse. p. 153. In Hazzard DG, Litz ML (eds): Symposium on Biological Effects and Characterization of Ultrasound Sources. Department of Health, Education and Welfare Publication No. FDA 78–8048. Government Printing Office, Washington, DC, 1977

39. Fry FJ, Erdmann WA, Johnson LK, et al: Ultrasonic Toxicity Study. Ultrasound Med Biol 3:35, 1978

40. Stolzenberg SJ, Torbit CA, Edmonds PD, et al: Effects of ultrasound on the mouse exposed at different stages of gestation: acute study. Radiat Environ Biophys 17:245, 1980

41. Stratmeyer ME: What do we know about the bioeffects. Presented at the 8th Annual National Conference on Radiation Control, May 2–7, Springfield, IL, 1976

42. Stratmeyer ME, Simmons LR, Pinkavitch FZ, et al: Growth and development of mice exposed in utero to ultrasound. p. 140. In Hazzard DG, Litz ML (eds): Symposium on Biological Effects and Characterizations of Ultrasound Sources. Department of Health, Education and Welfare Publication (FDA) 78–8048. Government Printing Office, Washington, DC, 1977

43. Sikov MR, Hildebrand BP, Sterns JD: Effects of exposure of nine-day rat embryo to Ultrasound. p. 529. In White DN, Barnes R (eds): Ultrasound in Medicine. Vol. 2. New York, 1976

8 Ultrasound and the Mammalian Fetus

EDWIN L. CARSTENSEN
ALLEN H. GATES

Almost all of the available information about the effects of ultrasound on the mammalian fetus comes through screening studies. Therein, the investigators have chosen one or more end-points, such as fetal weight, teratology, or behavioral characteristics, and compared these end-points for animals exposed to arbitrary ultrasonic fields with those of animals given a sham exposure (treated the same as exposed animals except that the ultrasound was not turned on). The choice of end-points in these studies has been determined more by the investigators' judgment of biological or clinical interest than by postulated mechanistic relationships between the physical agent, ultrasound, and biological effects. Among the numerous investigations on this subject, however, many different end-points have been selected.

The range of exposure conditions also has been very large. The rationale for the choice of exposure conditions has not been completely arbitrary. On the one hand, certain investigators have used clinical diagnostic ultrasound sources which in general have very low temporal-average intensities. On the other hand, most studies have been designed so that there is a reasonable chance of obtaining effects. Most investigators have been aware that ultrasound at sufficiently high average intensities will produce heat which, in turn, can have biological effects upon the fetus. As a consequence, it appears that, in the search for biological effects, many experiments were designed to reduce heating to "acceptable" but not necessarily negligible levels. It follows from this rationale in experimental design that many of the studies that report positive results have used exposure conditions that produce thermal effects or are on the borderline of producing them. Thus, for a critical analysis of the literature, one must consider the contribution which heat may have made to the claimed results.

LITERATURE SUMMARY

Negative Studies

It is interesting that more than half of the relevant studies on this subject are completely negative, that is, the investigations revealed no effects that could be attributed to ultrasound. Negative screening studies have relatively little scientific value. If experiments are not guided by rational postulates and the results are negative, it should not be assumed that they apply generally. It may be that the investigator simply was observing an insensitive end-point or was using either suboptimal exposure conditions or experimental procedures that were unable to detect subtle effects which actually were present.

It is relatively difficult to publish negative screening studies in reputable journals. Also, most investigators have a subtle bias toward finding results since it is neither personally nor scientifically rewarding to produce negative results over an extended period of time. Considering such factors, it is reassuring that this random searching, under exposure conditions (intensity and duration) which in many cases exceeded those typical of diagnostic procedures, revealed no marked deleterious effects.

It is noteworthy that none of approximately 15 clinical studies show significant effects. Possible exceptions include the report by David et al.[1] of increased fetal movement during exposure to ultrasound; however, related studies by Hertz and co-workers[2] and Powell-Phillips and Towell[3] failed to confirm those observations. Another possible exception is a retrospective analysis of clinical data which showed a small but statistically greater number of low birth weights among exposed than unexposed infants.[4] Since a large fraction of the referrals of patients for ultrasound relates to concern about fetal development, there may be an appreciable bias in selection of subjects for ultrasound diagnosis which could be reflected in birth weight.

It should be recognized that since there is little control over environmental influences to which subjects are exposed in epidemiologic surveys, this kind of study should be expected to reveal only large or unusual effects. Thus, even though the history of exposure of the human fetus to ultrasound is reassuring, clinical studies by their very nature would not necessarily reveal subtle or rare effects. Conversely, when an epidemiologic study shows a small but statistically significant correlation between some condition and exposure to ultrasound, that finding should be viewed cautiously until there is independent support in theory and laboratory studies.

Positive Claims

Those laboratory studies that have produced positive results are summarized in Table 8.1. The reports are listed in order of the increasing, minimum, temporal-average intensity required to produce an effect.

In certain studies, the sound was pulsed. For those cases, we have estimated the temporal peak intensity during the pulse. The definition of peak intensity is still in the process of refinement at the present time. Probably the best single predictor of transient cavitation is the maximum negative pressure in the pulse. Of the various definitions of peak intensity, the *maximum intensity* I_m (see Chapter 2) has the greatest relevance to known biological effects.[5, 6] Unfortunately, none of the studies reviewed here provide the detailed information necessary for a determination of I_m when the pulse lengths approach those used in diagnostic ultrasound. Hence, in Table 8.1, estimates of I_m are based on the rough concept that the temporal-average intensity (here labeled I^*) is just the product of I_m and the nominal pulse duration, multiplied by the pulse repetition rate. Whether the ultrasound is pulsed or not, the intensity varies in space and this must be recognized in specifying it. In the articles reviewed for Table 8.1, the intensity cited sometimes applied at a spatial peak and sometimes it was an average over a specified area; too often its nature was not explained. For the purposes of Table 8.1, the temporal-average intensities (whether spatial-average, spatial-peak or unknown) are taken as given in the reports, and are indicated as I^*.

For subtle effects in screening investigations, probably the best test of validity is confirmation by independent investigators. The status of each of the studies with regard to confirmation is indicated in the table. From the entire collection of studies, there is no clear consensus with regard to any biological effect.

FETAL WEIGHT

Perhaps the most intensively investigated end-point is fetal weight. As an illustration of the degree of consensus among investigators, we have summarized these results in Table 8.2. The study by Child et al.,[7] while a direct replicate of the report of Pizzarello and co-workers,[8] did not find the marked reductions in fetal weight at extremely low average intensities (I^*) and modest peak intensities (I_m) reported by the original authors. With the exception of the Pizzarello[8] and Muranaka[9] studies, the magnitudes of claimed effects on weight are small. Typical standard deviations for weights in sham (control) groups are of the order of 10 to 20 percent of the means. Most of the claimed weight changes are within that range. Although most of the studies listed cannot be compared directly, the possibility cannot be excluded that small reductions in fetal weight of mice and rats may result from exposures to intensities (I^*) of about 1–5 W/cm² for 2–5 minutes.

ULTRASONIC HEATING

Lele[10] definitively treated the question of heating in biomedical ultrasound. He concluded: (1) that, at certain states, the fetus is very sensitive to small elevations in temperature, and if fetal temperatures remain 2–5°C above normal for a few hours, increased congenital malformations result; and (2) that ultra-

TABLE 8.1 Summary of claimed positive effects of ultrasound upon the fetus[a]

Author	Effect	Frequency (MHz)	Minimum Surface Intensity (W/cm²)		Exposure Time (min)	Contact	H/V (cal/g)	Independent Confirmation
			I*	Im				
Pizzarello[8]	Decreased fetal weight in rats	2.2	0.001	1	5	Y	0.02	—
David[1]	Increased fetal movement in human subjects	—	0.01	—	15	Y	0.4	—
Rivers[22]	Growth retardation of chick embryos	2	0.01	P	3	—	0.1	0
Murai[23]	Behavior of rats: delay in maturation of grasp reflex	2.3	0.02		300	Y	20	0
Murai[24]	Behavior of rats: irradiated subjects showed more distinct vocalization in response to handling and more pronounced escape response from electroshock.	2.3	0.02	—	300	Y	20	0
Shimizu[25]	Skeletal malformations in mice	2.2	0.04		300	Y	38	+/−
Shoji[26]	Mortality in mice	2.25	0.04		300	Y	39	0
Shoji[27]	Prenatal death in mice	2.25	0.04		300	Y	39	0
Stratmeyer[28]	Lower body weight in mice	1	0.075		2	N	0.2	—
Muranaka[9]	Reduced fetal weight and increased fetal mortality in mice	2.3	0.1		4	—	1.3	+/−
Shoji[29]	Brain anomalies in rats	2.25	0.1		300	Y	97	0
Curto[30]	Increased postpartum mortality in mice	1	0.12	—	3	N	0.5	—
Stolzenberg[31]	Lower body weight in mice. Differences were noted only at 25 days of age.	2	0.5	—	3	N	4.3	+/−

Reference	End-point	Column 3	Column 4 (I*)	Column 5	Column 6	Column 7	Column 8	Column 9
Weinland[32]	Malformations in hamster embryos	1	0.5	—	2	Y	1.4	0
O'Brien[33]	Fetal weight reduction in mice	1	0.5	—	5	N	4	+/−
			5.5	—	0.2	—	2	
Takabayashi[21]	Increased weight in mice	2	0.6	60	5	N	8	0
Stratmeyer[34]	Increased weight in mice	1	0.75	—	2	N	2.3	—
Brettschneider[35]	Anomalies in chick embryos and frog eggs	0.8	1	—	10	—	11	0
Stolzenberg[36]	Fetal weight reduction and congenital malformations in mice	2	1	—	3.3	N	10	+/−
Mannor[37]	Small fetuses and fetal death in mice	2.3	1	—	15	N	50	0
Rugh[38]	Teratogenic effects in mice	1	2	—	3	N	9	0
Taylor[19]	Increased congenital abnormalities in chick embryos	1	2.5	25	5	N	18	0
Sikov[16]	Fetal death and malformations	0.7	6	—	5	N	30	0
		3.2	10	—	5	—	230	0
Fry[18]	Effects in mice. Decreased litter size. Early and late resorptions. Increased anomalies. Decreased fetal weight	1.4	45	1,900	0.5	N	45	0

ªColumn 1 gives the senior author of the study. Column 2 lists the end-point of the study and gives the experimental animal used. Column 3 is the nominal frequency. Of course, with very short pulses the radiation actually involves a spectrum about the nominal frequency. At the highest peak intensities, the radiation contains nonlinearly generated harmonics of the nominal frequency. Column 4 gives the temporal-average intensity (I*), discussed in the text. With pulsed sources, Column 5 provides an estimate of the maximum intensity I_m as defined in the text. Column 6 is the exposure duration. Column 7 indicates whether the transducer was in direct contact with the animal (Y) or whether contact was made through a fluid couplant (N). In the latter case, the animal frequently was mounted in a water tank which served to facilitate heat exchange. Column 8 is the nominal absorbed energy per unit volume given in calories per cubic centimeter (the product of twice the absorption coefficient of the tissue, and temporal-average intensity (I*) and the exposure time divided by 4.2). Column 9 indicates whether the observation has been confirmed by independent investigators (+), whether replicate or similar studies failed to confirm the observations (−), or whether no attempt has as yet been made to confirm the work (0).

TABLE 8.2 Effects of ultrasound upon fetal weight[a]

Author	Intensity (W/cm²) I*	Intensity (W/cm²) I_m	Exposure Time (min)	Change in Fetal Weight (%)
Pizzarello[8]	0.001	1	5	−50
McClain[39]	0.01	—	120	(No effect)
Child[7]	0.015	12	5	(No effect)
Murai[24]	0.02	—	300	(No effect)
Stratmeyer[34]	0.08	—	2	+9
Muranaka[9]	0.1	—	4	−50
Stolzenberg[31]	0.5	—	3	−8
Takabayashi[21]	0.6	60	5	(No effect)
Stratmeyer[28]	0.8	—	2	−2
Sikov[40]	1	—	5	(No effect)
Stolzenberg[36]	1	—	3	−8
Kimmel[41]	1	—	2	(No effect)
O'Brien[42]	2.5	—	0.3	(No effect)
Kim[43]	2.5	—	0.3	(No effect)
O'Brien[33]	5.5	—	0.2	−10
Sikov[44]	10	—	5	(No effect)
Warwick[17]	27	490	0.4	(No effect)
Fry[18]	51	1,900	0.3	−19

[a] Studies are listed in order of increasing temporal-average intensity (I*). Standard deviations for fetal weights reported by various investigators fall in the range of 10–20 percent of the mean value for sham-exposed animals.

sonic heating in almost any practical, diagnostic application of ultrasound in obstetrics is far too small to cause teratologic effects. This is consistent with the estimations of ultrasonic heating by Nyborg and Steele[11] if realistic values of exposure parameters are assumed. Although we do not have a complete assessment of the average intensities which characterize obstetric practice, enough is known[12, 13] (Appendix A) to assure us that we can ignore heat as a mechanism of concern in evaluation of potential hazards in all obstetric applications of pulsed ultrasound and probably in most uses of continuous-wave (CW) Doppler devices. On the contrary, this cannot be done when evaluating many of the experimental studies of the effects of ultrasound on laboratory animal fetuses.

To emphasize this latter point, Table 8.1 contains a column (H/V) giving the total heat per unit volume generated by the exposure. This is simply the product of twice the absorption coefficient of the tissue, the temporal-average intensity (I*) and the time (in seconds), divided by 4.2, and is expressed in calories per cubic centimeter. We have taken the absorption coefficient to be

0.05 f cm^{-1}, where f is the frequency in megahertz. Assuming no loss of heat by convection or conduction during the treatment, this number would approximate the temperature elevation in degrees Centigrade. Because the cooling effect of blood perfusion is not taken into account, this is a very conservative upper boundary for the actual temperature rise in the experiment. However, inspection of the (H/V) column in Table 8.1 shows that there are very few confirmed experiments that report positive results where a role for heat can be clearly ruled out.

PULSED ULTRASOUND

From the above discussion and the data available in Tables 8.1 and 8.2, it appears doubtful that any effects on the animal fetus have been demonstrated from exposures to CW ultrasound which were not, at least in part, influenced by the heat generated by absorption of the radiation or by conduction of heat from the transducer. Yet, heat is not a factor in most diagnostic uses of ultrasound in obstetrics. It follows that there is nothing in the literature on exposures of the fetus to CW ultrasound to indicate clearly that any hazards are to be expected in the normal obstetric use of ultrasound.

Although heat is not a mechanism of concern in obstetrical ultrasound, we cannot be as complacent with regard to cavitation. Flynn[14] has shown that if appropriate nuclei are present, transient cavitation may be induced even with diagnostic, microsecond-length pulses.[15]

Two conditions are required for transient cavitation: (1) peak intensities exceeding 2–50 W/cm^2 depending upon frequency,[15] and (2) the existence of appropriate nuclei. Many pulse-echo units in use today exceed these thresholds. Whether gas bodies of appropriate size exist in close proximity to the fetus is a difficult question to assess. There are no direct methods for detection of the bubbles in vivo.

Normally, bubbles of submicron size in pure water would be unstable and, if created, would be dissolved. Yet, the very existence of transient cavitation at modest intensities demonstrates that bubbles can be stabilized. It is very likely that if cavitation nuclei exist at all near the fetus, they are rare, and that if cavitation-related effects occurred, they would be difficult to detect.

There is no clear evidence in the studies which have been summarized in Table 8.1 to support the suggestion that cavitation affects the fetus. Maximum intensities (I_m) in several studies exceed the threshold for transient cavitation by a wide margin. But because of variability in location of cavitation nuclei and in susceptibility of the fetus, we expect that any clues from studies of effects on the fetus will be elusive. At one time, Sikov and Hildebrand[16] observed an increase in cardiac defects as I_m approached 100 W/cm^2; they were not able to replicate the observations in subsequent work. Out of a very large study, Warwick et al.[17] found one set of exposure conditions (I_m = 225 W/cm^2 repeated on 5 different days of gestation) which produced significantly increased rates of abnormalities among the fetuses; however, that particular group of animals was dominated by 6 abnormal fetuses from a single female parent. Fry et al.[18] used a broad beam in which I_m was 600 W/cm² and a narrow beam in which I_m was 1,900 W/cm² to expose the mouse uterus in such a way that the product of intensity and time for the tissue was approximately the same; effects on the fetuses (litter size, resorptions, and fetal anomalies) were greater at the higher intensity than they were at the lower intensity. Taylor and Dyson[19] found increased anomalies in chick embryos after in vitro exposure to maximum intensities (I_m) of 25 W/cm² and 40 W/cm² but not with maximum intensities of 10 W/cm². These numbers are similar to those found to be lethal to *Drosophila* larvae.[20] Finally, Takabayashi et al.[21] reported increased anomalies in mice after exposures in utero to maximum intensities (I_m) of 60 W/cm². It was necessary for the authors to base their conclusions on two unreplicated experiments, but their observations are consistent with a conclusion that the threshold for anomalies is near 60 W/cm² for I_m and requires pulse lengths on the order of 5–10 μsec.

CONCLUSIONS AND RECOMMENDATIONS

Diagnostic ultrasound, as with any other agent, cannot be proven absolutely safe. In practice, for any medical or environmental exposure, an operational definition of safety is used, namely, the absence of identifiable hazards. With this in mind, we have surveyed the available information relative to exposure of the fetus. This may be one of the most sensitive ages in mammals wherein damage to a few cells at certain stages of development may be multiplied to gross effects as the conceptus develops. The clinical importance of the safety question is difficult to overestimate. However, in terms of identifiable effects on the exposed fetus, pulse-echo ultrasound as used in obstetrics has not been proven hazardous.

Nevertheless, a responsible and vigilant scientific community will continue the search for effects. Interestingly, developments in the theory of cavitation,[14, 15] together with the experimental observations of pronounced deleterious effects at diagnostic levels of pulsed ultrasound on *Drosophila* larvae[20] give a new impetus to that search. In this review of the literature, we find hints of possible effects with pulsed ultrasound at levels that exceed the theoretical threshold for transient cavitation. Innovative concepts in experimental design are needed to further elucidate the subject. Care should be taken to be certain that the influence of heat does not inadvertently obscure the observation of important nonthermal phenomena in future studies of the biological effects of pulsed ultrasound.

Available information indicates that there are thresholds for transient cavitation which are on the order of 10 W/cm² for I_m in microsecond-length pulses. It should be possible to perform almost all of the diagnostic procedures in obstetrics with maximum intensities substantially below these levels.

A clinician who wishes to be conservative may choose to use I_m levels below 10 W/cm², unless information obtainable only at higher intensities justifies exceeding that level. However, at present, the clinician would be restricted in the choice of equipment because only a few manufacturers make the required intensity data conveniently available. All manufacturers should include acoustic output information in technical specifications for their equipment to aid the obstetrician in planning the procedures to be used.

ACKNOWLEDGMENTS

The authors are indebted to Dr. Peter Edmonds and Dr. Mel Stratmeyer for data and helpful discussions. Mrs. Sally Child provided help and guidance during the preparation of this chapter.

This study was supported in part by United States Public Health Service Grants GM09933 and ES01247.

A more complete review of this subject has been prepared as an internal report No. GM09933-21 entitled "Effects of Ultrasound on the Fetus." Copies of this report can be supplied upon request.

REFERENCES

1. David H, Weaver JB, Pearson JF: Doppler ultrasound and fetal activity. Br Med J 2:62, 1975
2. Hertz RH, Timor-Tritsch I, Dierker LJ, Jr, et al: Continuous ultrasound and fetal movement. Am J Obstet Gynecol 135:152, 1975
3. Powell-Phillips WD, Towell ME: Doppler ultrasound and subjective assessment of fetal activity. Br Med J 2:101, 1979
4. Moore RM, Jr, Barrick KM, Hamilton TM: Effect of sonic radiation on growth and development. Proceedings of the Meeting of the Society for Epidemiologic Research, Cincinnati, OH, June 16–18, 1982
5. Carstensen EL, Parker KJ, Barbee DB: Temporal peak intensity. J Acoust Soc Am 74:1057, 1983
6. Carstensen EL, Berg RB, Child SZ: Pulse average vs maximum intensity. Ultrasound Med Biol 9:L451, 1983
7. Child SZ, Davis H, Carstensen EL: A test for the effects of low-temporal-average-intensity, pulsed ultrasound on the rat fetus. Exp Cell Biol 52:207, 1984
8. Pizzarello DJ, Vivino A, Maden B, et al: Effect of pulsed low-power ultrasound on growing tissues. Exp Cell Biol 46:179, 1978
9. Muranaka A, Tachibana M, Suzuki F: Effects of ultrasound on embryonic development and fetal growth in mice. Teratology 10:91, 1974 (abstr)
10. Lele PP: Ultrasonic teratology in mouse and man. p. 22. In Proceedings 2nd European Congress on Ultrasonics in Medicine, Excerpta Medica Int Cong Ser No. 363. Excerpta Medica, Amsterdam-Oxford, 1975
11. Nyborg WL, Steele RB: Temperature elevation in a beam of ultrasound. Ultrasound Med Biol 9:611, 1983
12. Stewart HF: Output levels from commercial, diagnostic ultrasound equipment. Presented at the Fall Meeting of the American Institute of Ultrasound Medicine, New York, October 1983
13. National Council on Radiation Protection and Measurements (NCRP): Biological Effects of Ultrasound: Mechanisms and Clinical Applications. NCRP Report No. 74. NCRP Publications, Bethesda, MD
14. Flynn HG: Generation of transient cavities in liquids by microsecond pulses of ultrasound. J Acoust Soc Am 72:1926, 1982
15. Carstensen EL, Flynn HG: The potential for transient cavitation with microsecond pulses of ultrasound. Ultrasound Med Biol 8:L720, 1982

16. Sikov MR, Hildebrand BP: Effects of prenatal exposure to ultrasound. p. 267. In Persaud TVN (ed): Advances in the Study of Birth Defects. Vol. 2. Teratological Testing. MTP Press Ltd, International Medical Publ, Falcon House, Lancaster, England, 1979

17. Warwick R, Pond JB, Woodward B, Connolly CC: Hazards of diagnostic ultrasonography—a study with mice. IEEE Trans Sonics Ultrasonics SU-17:158, 1970

18. Fry FJ, Erdmann WA, Johnson LK, Baird AI: Ultrasonic toxicity study. Ultrasound Med Biol 3:351, 1978

19. Taylor KJW, Dyson M: Toxicity studies on the interaction of ultrasound on embryonic and adult tissues. p. 353. In Ultrasonics in Medicine (Proceedings 2nd World Congress Ultrasound in Medicine). Excerpta Medica, Amsterdam, 1973

20. Child SZ, Carstensen EL, Lam SK: Effects of ultrasound on *Drosophila:* III. Exposure of larvae to low-temporal-average-intensity, pulsed irradiation. Ultrasound Med Biol 7:167, 1981

21. Takabayashi T, Abe Y, Sato S, Suzuki M: Effects of pulse-wave ultrasonic irradiation on mouse embryo. Cho-Onpa Igaku (Med Ultrasound) 8:286, 1981

22. Rivers DB, Elmer WA, Rehfield LW: Changes in the rate of development of chick embryos subject to diagnostic pulsed ultrasound. p. 20. In Proceedings 17th Annual Meeting American Institute of Ultrasound in Medicine 1972, Philadelphia: October 29, 1972

23. Murai N, Hoshi K, Nakamura T: Effects of diagnostic ultrasound irradiated during fetal stage on development of orienting behavior and reflex ontogeny in rats. Tohoku J Exp Med 116:17, 1975

24. Murai N, Hoshi K, Kang C, Suzuki M: Effects of diagnostic ultrasound irradiated during foetal stage on emotional and cognitive behavior in rats. Tohoku J Exp Med 117:225, 1975

25. Shimizu T, Shoji R: An experimental safety study of mice exposed to low-intensity ultrasound. Excerpta Medica Int Ser 277:28, 1973

26. Shoji R, Momma E, Shimizu T, Matsuda S: An experimental study on the effect of low-intensity ultrasound on developing mouse embryos. J Fac Sci Hokkaido U, Ser VI 18:51, 1971

27. Shoji R, Murakami U, Shimizu T: Influence of low-intensity ultrasonic irradiation on prenatal development of two inbred mouse strains. Teratology 12:227, 1975

28. Stratmeyer ME, Pinkavitch FZ, Simmons LR, Sternthal P: *In utero* effects of ultrasound exposure in mice. 26th Annual Meeting American Institute of Ultrasound in Medicine and 10th Annual Meeting Society Diagnostic Medical Sonography, San Francisco, August 17–21, 1981

29. Shoji R, Murakami U: Further studies on the effect of ultrasound on mouse and rat embryos. Teratology 10:97, 1974

30. Curto KA: Early postpartum mortality following ultrasound radiation. Ultrasound Med 2:535, 1976

31. Stolzenberg SJ, Torbit CA, Pryor GT, Edmonds PD: Toxicity of ultrasound in mice: neonatal studies. Radiat Environ Biophys 18:37, 1980

32. Weinland LS: Production of abnormal hamster embryos with ultrasound. Penn Acad Sci 37:48, 1963

33. O'Brien WD, Dose dependent effect of ultrasound on fetal weight in mice. J Ultrasound Med 2:1, 1983

34. Stratmeyer ME, Simmons LR, Pinkavitch FZ, et al: Growth and development of mice exposed *in utero* to ultrasound. p. 140. In Symposium on Biological Effects and Characterization of Ultrasonic Sources. Department of Health, Education and Welfare Publication (FDA) 78–8148. Bethesda, Md, 1977

35. Brettschneider H: Die Wirking der Ultraschalls auf die Entwicklung des Hunchens und des Froscheis. Strahlentherapie 87:517, 1952

36. Stolzenberg SJ, Torbit CA, Edmonds PD, Tanzer JC: Effects of ultrasound on the mouse exposed at different stages of gestation: acute studies. Radiat Environ Biophys 18:245, 1980

37. Mannor SM, Serr DM, Tamari I, et al: The safety of ultrasound in fetal monitoring. Am J Obstet Gynecol 113:653, 1972

38. Rugh R, McManaway M: Can ultrasound be teratogenic? p. 175. In Symposium on Biological Effects and Characterization of Ultrasonic Sources. Department of Health, Education and Welfare Publication (FDA) 78–8148. Bethesda, Md, 1977

39. McClain RM, Hoar RM, Saltzman MB: Teratology study of rats exposed to ultrasound. J Obstet Gynecol 14:39, 1972

40. Sikov MR, Collins DH: Embryotoxic potential of cw ultrasound in the preimplantation rat embryo. J Ultrasound Med, suppl., 1:141, 1982

41. Kimmel CH, Stratmeyer ME, Galloway WD, et al: An evaluation of the teratogenic potential of ultrasound exposure in pregnant ICR mice. 26th Annual Meeting American Institute of Ultrasound in Medicine and 10th Annual Meeting Society of Diagnostic Sonography, San Francisco, August 17–21, 1981

42. O'Brien WD, Jr, Januzik SJ, Dunn F: Ultrasound biologic effects: a suggestion of strain specificity. J Ultrasound Med 1:367, 1982

43. Kim HKL, Picciano MF, O'Brien WD, Jr: The combined effect of ultrasonic exposure and protein restriction on maternal and fetal mice. Ultrasound Med Biol 9:165, 1983

44. Sikov MR, Hildebrand BP: Effects of ultrasound on the prenatal development of the rat. Part 1. 3.2 MHz continuous wave at nine days of gestation. J Clin Ultrasound 4:357, 1976

9 The Use of Diagnostic Ultrasound on the Human Fetus

CHARLES W. HOHLER

The purpose of this chapter is to discuss the applications of diagnostic ultrasound in obstetrics with special attention to how our knowledge of biological effects of ultrasound influences such use. The immediate major benefits derived from having the unique diagnostic information made possible only by fetal exposure to diagnostic ultrasound, often have a major impact on subsequent pregnancy management. In fact, use of diagnostic ultrasound in obstetrics is currently mainly restricted to those clinical situations where management decisions require direct information about fetal status. No other imaging technique currently available can replace or rival the capabilities of diagnostic ultrasound for rapid provision of diagnostically efficacious information.

Enthusiasm for the remarkable diagnostic information which can be obtained using diagnostic ultrasound may have, in the past, overshadowed concerns on the part of some clinicians about the possibility of adverse biological effects of ultrasound on the developing fetus and embryo. However, this situation is beginning to change.

Heightened awareness, on the part of patients, physicians, professional organizations, and manufacturers, as well as greater governmental activity in promoting investigation into the interaction of ultrasound energy with biological tissues, over the past few years, have all lead to the present state of interest in (and in many cases, understandable confusion over) the complex and often contradictory ultrasound bioeffects literature.

Some have looked at the lack of acute effects of diagnostic ultrasound on the fetus as evidence of the benign nature of such fetal exposure. However, this "empirical" safety record of use of both pulsed and continuous-wave ultrasound in obstetrics should not leave the clinician complacent about biological effects. It is unlikely that subtle, long-term, biological effects, if any, of diagnostic ultrasound exposure on the fetus would be appreciated in this manner. The only statement that can be made on the basis of such clinical observations is that diagnostic ultrasound use in pregnancy does not appear to represent an acute material and significant hazard to the fetus. Whether the concern about theoretical long-term bioeffects from fetal exposure to diagnostic ultrasound is justified or not remains to be seen.

In the meantime, it would be wise to view all extreme interpretations of the available experimental literature with caution, if not skepticism. In some cases, failure to appreciate this caveat can lead to physician overreaction and consequent unnecessary patient anxiety. This is indeed unfortunate. Due to the complexity of the analysis required to properly evaluate both experimental design and end-points used to study the biological effects of ultrasound, the average physician (let alone even the most responsible television and print report) often finds it difficult to put into proper perspective new data as they are published. Furthermore, there are some self-appointed "experts" who are provoking great media attention and generating unfair patient anxiety by selective, and in some cases irresponsible interpretation of the bioeffects literature. This has had predictable consequences on clinical patient care. Curiosity and interest has often turned into irrational concern on the part of both physicians and patients, who may be led to illogical insistence on a "zero risk" for medical procedures. Unfortunately, if one is told often enough that something is harmful, then the preception of harm may be just as detrimental to patient well-being, as if the perception were indeed the reality.

The reality is that there does exist a large body of bioeffects literature which is negative and reassuring. However, some of the literature suggests that adverse fetal biological effects of ultrasound exposure can occur, at what would be considered "diagnostic" intensities. Even allowing for poor dosimetry, lack of confirmation of many studies, and difficulty in extrapolation to the human situation from animal data, it is becoming increasingly apparent that the safety of fetal diagnostic ultrasound exposure should be looked upon as only a relative condition. Heat and cavitation effects can perhaps explain most of the positive results to date, but basic scientific investigations into possible effects of ultrasound exposure on fetal cell development, microarchitecture, tissue organization and function, protein production, and cell division, remain, for the most part, unexplored in an organized, systematic way.

Faced with such uncertainty the prudent clinician is faced with a dilemma. Clear-cut benefits exist from use of ultrasound. In some cases, the diagnostic information obtained means life or death for the developing fetus. The immediate risk to the fetus from failure to make a timely diagnosis by application of ultrasound may present a clear and present danger of far greater moment than any conceivable long-term theoretical risk to well-being in the future.

Nevertheless, the possibility of unknown (unrecognized?) risks dictates a cautious approach to utilization of diagnostic ultrasound, no matter what the perceived benefits may be. Prudence, however, should not be replaced by nihilism. The recognized benefits of use of diagnostic ultrasound in the modern practice of obstetrics are real and present, both for the family and the developing fetus. Even the presence of a "negative" result from an ultrasound examination is important information for both the family and the physician to possess. The dangers, if any, on the other hand, still remain theoretical.

We would probably do well to anticipate that some form of adverse biological effect may be found in the future. It would almost be better in some ways if that were to happen. Because, then, we would have a true benefit versus risk equation to consider. Now, we really don't. But, if the clinician were to approach each proposed ultrasound examination in pregnancy AS IF there were demonstrated adverse biological effects on the fetus and/or mother from diagnostic ultrasound use, then he would be forced to weigh the impact on further pregnancy management of the information gained from each ultrasound exposure.

The question of "informed consent" also comes up quite often in the clinical setting. If there were a demonstrated "material risk" to the use of ultrasound in pregnancy, then it would be necessary to obtain such consent. Where no material risk is demonstrable, then it is not necessary to do so. In the author's laboratory, no such consent is obtained for routine antepartum and intrapartum obstetrical ultrasound examinations.

To create an enlightened public understanding of the emerging critical role of diagnostic ultrasound in obstetrics as it is currently practiced, will require much time and effort. Patients need to appreciate that application of ultrasound in obstetrics, like much of medicine, is not an exact science. Benefits and risks should be carefully and completely explained to patients who express a desire to know. Certain other situations (e.g., where physician philosophy concerning use of ultrasound may lead to ultrasound exposure with as yet unproven direct fetal or maternal benefit, such as the routine screening of all pregnant patients) should lead to full disclosure to patients, in order to give them the opportunity to refuse such examinations if they so desire. It needs to be reinforced that we physicians apply our medical skills for the benefit of our patients based on our understanding of the risks and benefits as we perceive them from formal and continuing medical education. On the clinician's part, compassionate understanding of the public dilemma posed by our professional uncertainty must continue to be shown to our patients. It is easy to understand how that concern can so easily be aroused by widely publicized, self-styled experts often conveying a selective reading of the bioeffects literature, when we ourselves share the same kinds of concerns. Finally, it is our duty to display, at all times, a candid willingness to discuss these issues with our patients and to keep an open mind to new data as they appear. All of these factors will, it is hoped, lead to more rapid clarification of the ultimate role of diagnostic ultrasound in obstetrics. The following discussion should be read with that perspective firmly in mind.

THE ROLE OF OBSTETRIC ULTRASOUND TODAY

The introduction of the dynamic-imaging real-time linear-array into clinical obstetric diagnosis in the United States in 1974, heralded the beginning of a quiet revolution in obstetric patient care and fetal surveillance which continues unabated to the present day. Diagnostic ultrasound, especially dynamic-imag-

TABLE 9.1 Current obstetric uses of diagnostic ultrasound that are of proven efficacy in the human

Estimation of gestational age
Fetal weight estimation and serial observation of fetal growth
Detection of fetal life
Pregnancy location determination
Placenta localization
Estimation of amniotic fluid volume
Determination of fetal number and presentation
Evaluation of threatened abortion
Ovarian follicle development serial observation
Diagnosis of hydatidiform mole
IUD localization in pregnancy
Detection of uterine leiomyomata and pelvic masses
Detection of certain types of structural and functional congenital defects
Adjunctive use to assist needle placement for amniocentesis and intrauterine transfusions

Abbreviations: IUD, intrauterine device.

ing, is emerging as a unique diagnostic tool of unequaled economy, convenience, and efficacy. Few technologic developments have sparked the imagination of clinicians and laypersons alike, as has the application of ultrasound energy to fetal observation.

Over the past 25 years, diagnostic ultrasound has gone from a research tool to such a commonly used clinical technology that it is currently estimated that one third of obstetricians have diagnostic ultrasound equipment in their offices and clinics.[1] Over half of all pregnant women receive at least one diagnostic ultrasound examination, especially women in whom pregnancy is considered "high risk" (i.e., in which medical complications are seen to exist which might interfere with normal fetal growth and development). The major current uses of diagnostic ultrasound in obstetrics that are of *proven* benefit are listed in Table 9.1.

In the present context, it is important for the informed clinician to understand where diagnostic ultrasound has been found to be of proven benefit in leading

TABLE 9.2 Current uses of obstetric ultrasound that are of probable benefit in the human

Postpartum uterus evaluation
Intrapartum obstetric uses
Biophysical profile assessment of fetal well-being

TABLE 9.3 Investigational uses of obstetric ultrasound in the human

Intrauterine shunt placement guidance for fetal surgery

Fetal echocardiography

Postdates pregnancy evaluation

Adjunct to external version of breech presentation

Doppler blood flow studies of the placental and fetal circulation

to improvement of reproductive outcome, and where such strong evidence is sparse or even lacking. When possible, references which document the efficacy of ultrasound applications are provided. From the following discussion, it will be seen that it appears that the future applications of this technology will be limited only by the human imagination and by the available ultrasound equipment, plus computer technology provided for clinical use.

Besides those of proven value, there are areas of obstetrics and gynecology in which the use of diagnostic ultrasound is felt to be of benefit by many investigators, but strong scientific evidence of such efficacy has not yet been forthcoming. Such uses that are of probable benefit are listed in Table 9.2. In many of these applications, such use is so new that the relative benefits, costs, and risks of such use vis-à-vis other imaging or diagnostic modalities remain to be completely assessed. Major areas of active clinical investigation are listed in Table 9.3.

The four major applications of diagnostic ultrasound in obstetrics will each be discussed to highlight the wide range of uses to which this energy has been put. They are: (1) pregnancy dating, (2) fetal growth evaluation, (3) detection of congenital structural anomalies, and (4) assessment of fetal well-being. These general areas of utilization are the broadest, but it should be recognized by the reader that they are by no means the only ones that are of importance in present clinical practice.

PREGNANCY DATING

Estimation of gestational age is one of the cornerstones of obstetrical prenatal care. Clinical methods of pregnancy dating become somewhat less accurate as gestation progresses,[2-10] especially when confounding factors are found to exist. Clinical pregnancy dating becomes less reliable than ultrasound dating in the face of such common complicating factors as the patient's inability to recall the starting date of the last menstrual period (LMP) correctly, the use of oral contraceptives, lactation, patient obesity, the presence of uterine leiomyomata, the common necessity of having multiple physicians examine the patient at different gestational ages, and the subjective nature of maternal reporting of quickening. Approximately two thirds of all examination requests in our laboratory are for this indication.

Ultrasound pregnancy dating has been shown to be both accurate and precise, and better clinically for assigning gestational age in the presence of the above complications, than has any other available method. Gestational sac mean diameter and volume and the crown-rump length (CRL) of the fetus are the primary ultrasound dating methods used prior to the 13th week of gestation (from the first day of the LMP). Pregnancy dating by use of the CRL is accurate to plus or minus 5–7 days in approximately 95 percent of cases. Recently, it has been shown that the percentage of patients who deliver within 7 days of the ultrasound-predicted estimated date of delivery (EDD), by either CRL measurement or by a biparietal diameter (BPD) measurement between 13 and 20 weeks, is equivalent.[11]

Because of a presumption that the period of fetal organogenesis is the most vulnerable to ultrasound exposure, the above finding is important from the biological effects viewpoint. It means that it is feasible to delay ultrasound dating until after the first trimester without sacrifice of either accuracy or precision for this task. Furthermore, there appear to be additional benefits to this delay, in that fetal anatomy becomes more easily recognizable after the 16th week of gestation. The 16- to 20-week time period for fetal gestational age estimation, is the primary time for other forms of prenatal diagnosis, such as amniocentesis on women of age 35 at increased risk for chromosomal anomalies such as trisomy 21 and for serum α-fetoprotein (AFP) determinations which are used to detect fetal neural tube defects. Furthermore, anatomic landmarks can be seen well, because of the relatively large amount of amniotic fluid present surrounding the fetus.

Fetal cephalometry has been the most widely used method for pregnancy dating—after 12 completed weeks of gestation. At first, in the 1960s, using bistable static B-scanners, the "line" of the falx cerebrum could be visualized to properly align BPD measurements, but virtually no other internal intracranial anatomy could be seen. Later, in the mid-1970s, the gray-scaling of B-scan images (after development of the electronic scan converter) gave a new look to the fetal head. The wealth of anatomic detail confused observers and put into question the validity of BPD growth curves developed on more primitive equipment. At the same time, some degree of standardization of measurement planes and landmarks, as well as techniques, has occurred with consequent improvement in proper assignment of gestational age using this parameter.[12-16] Nevertheless, it is generally agreed that the variation in BPD size at any given gestational age becomes greater as pregnancy progresses. Optimally, measurement of fetal BPD should be done before 26 weeks (and preferably prior to 20 weeks). If a single, technically good measurement of the BPD agrees to within 1 week of the best clinical estimate of dates, then it appears that no alteration of the estimated date of delivery needs to be done. If, however, there is more than 1 week difference between the two estimates, the ultrasound BPD-estimated EDD should be used. Many clinicians prefer to follow up this examination with another several weeks later to watch fetal growth after such a reassignment of gestational age, in order not to miss a possible subtle beginning of intrauterine growth retardation (IUGR) which began early in gestation.

Many growth curves for the BPD have been published. They are all quite similar.[17-20] When the BPD cannot be measured or when temporary, position-related fetal head shape changes occur in utero, then alternative pregnancy dating methods, such as measurement of fetal head circumference (HC), abdomen circumference (AC), or femur length, can all be used together or individually, to estimate age without sacrifice of precision or accuracy. Under certain conditions (such as with multiple gestation) or with certain coexistent maternal medical complications of pregnancy (such as diabetes mellitus, chronic renal disease, or hypertension), such alternative measurements may relate more closely to fetal size than gestational age. Much work remains to define the proper roles for all of these measurements for pregnancy dating in relation to the measurement of the BPD. Early on, however, it has become obvious that many fetal measurements can effectively take the place of the historically, more well accepted, BPD measurements in order to accurately judge gestational age with diagnostic ultrasound.[21-26]

FETAL GROWTH RETARDATION

A second major application of diagnostic ultrasound is monitoring of fetal growth rates between exams and to estimate fetal weight for dates. Thus, accurate pregnancy dating is essential for ultrasound fetal measurements to describe how any given fetus compares to its peers at each gestational age. Clinically, knowledge of weight-for-dates has been shown to bear directly on pregnancy outcome.[27-30] Intrauterine growth delay or retardation can occur for a variety of complex reasons, either due to *intrinsic* fetal congenital anomalies or viral infections, or it can be due to *extrinsic* causes related, primarily, to chronic fetal undernutrition secondary to chronic reduction in placental perfusion with well-oxygenated blood.

The goals of ultrasound monitoring of fetal growth are several: (1) to improve upon the 50 percent clinical detection rate for IUGR, (2) to monitor the severity and progression of the disorder, and (3) to determine, if possible, the etiology of the disorder.

Fortunately, the same measurements used for pregnancy dating can also be used to assess fetal size and body symmetry. This last is important, since different fetal organs have been found to respond to a different degree and at different rates to the same growth retarding influence. Head circumference and AC are used indirectly to measure fetal brain and liver weights, respectively, while using the BPD and AC to determine fetal weight.[31-34]

Of the abnormal growth patterns detectable with diagnostic ultrasound, IUGR is of most concern, because a significant number of these fetuses will be stillborn or have long-term neurologic sequelae, which are now preventable through early ultrasound growth failure detection and antenatal biophysical fetal surveillance. Biparietal diameter measurement alone, however, has been shown to be relatively insensitive as a "screening" method for the presence of IUGR by most, but not all, investigators.[35-37]

Macrosomia is also detectable. The obese fetus with more than ample liver glycogen stores is detected by comparison of head and abdomen circumferences.

The HC/AC ratio will be low and the estimated fetal weight will be greater than the ninetieth percentile when macrosomia is present. This use of the HC/AC ratio is the converse of the original use for the detection of depleted liver glycogen stores which would indicate the presence of IUGR.[38, 39] However, this use is effective, though the ability to detect with great accuracy the fetus that will weigh more than 4,000 g at birth still remains elusive. Thus, shoulder dystocia in these large babies remains a major obstetric problem.[40]

The use of ultrasound to detect fetal growth abnormalities is best applied in the last half of pregnancy, when chronic uteroplacental insufficiency becomes clinically manifest. Early confirmation of clinical dates makes this later evaluation of fetal growth much more exact and/or possible. While serial ultrasound examinations are not usually necessary for pregnancy dating, the plotting of individual fetal growth profiles against established normal weight-for-dates curves,[41-43] when medical complications of pregnancy are present, is essential to optimal obstetric care. On the basis of a single ultrasound examination performed in the third trimester, little can be said about pregnancy dating, although an estimate of weight and body proportions can be effectively made, when medical complications of pregnancy or known congenital abnormalities of the fetus are present which might interfere with normal fetal growth.

It should be kept in mind that the definition of IUGR and of macrosomia are statistical definitions and are, therefore, somewhat arbitrary methods of fetal growth evaluation that, in many cases, are incomplete. Not all babies growing below the 10th percentile or above the 90th percentile are abnormal, nor are all babies growing between the 10th and 90th percentiles normal. Other methods of fetal growth evaluation, such as the Ponderal index,[44, 45] may afford a better separation of the well-nourished from the malnourished fetus.

Use of diagnostic ultrasound for fetal growth evaluation illustrates several accepted biological principles: (1) The uterus can sometimes become a rather "hostile" environment for the developing fetus; (2) different fetal organs respond to insults secondary to poor or chronically reduced placental perfusion, to a different extent and at different rates; and (3) brain size, body length, and body weight of the fetus all must be measured to adequately profile fetal growth in utero, before a definitive ultrasound diagnosis can be entertained. Without such careful analysis, many false-positive and false-negative diagnoses of IUGR or macrosomia will be the result.

CONGENITAL STRUCTURAL ANOMALY DETECTION

With high-resolution ultrasound equipment currently available, it is now possible to diagnose many fetal structural anomalies in the second and third trimesters of pregnancy. Abnormalities of the fetal skull and brain, chest contents, abdomen, kidneys, bladder, bowel, and limbs can all be identified. Such information, when coupled with increasingly sophisticated information from the results of genetic amniocentesis for karyotype, AFP, and acetylcholinesterase determinations, can lead to specific diagnoses for the fetus at risk. In the second trimester of pregnancy, this is important so that patients can be offered a choice of alternative managements; while in the third trimester, patients and their physicians can better manage diagnosed fetal anomalies, such that affected babies can be born or treated in utero at the right time and delivered at the right location, with the right support team and equipment available, such that functional and anatomical deficits can be minimized.

Approximately 20 percent of patients with hydramnios have an anomalous fetus.[46] Precise determination of amniotic fluid volume is not possible with routine diagnostic ultrasound techniques. Polyhydramnios can be caused by anomalies related to fetal inability to swallow, as well as fetal bowel obstruction proximal to the ileum. Diaphragmatic hernia can also be found when polyhydramnios is present. However, this is not an invariable finding. Sometimes, fetal hydrops or ascites is present secondary to fetal cardiac failure, venous obstruction, hypoproteinemia, or immune sensitization. Occasionally, this is found to be transient. The thickened placenta associated with severe hydrops from Rh sensitization or other nonimmune conditions can also be visualized.

In conjunction with serum AFP screening, diagnostic ultrasound is used to detect fetal neural tube defects, such as anencephaly, spina bifida, and meningomyelocele. Two to 3 percent of pregnancies from AFP screening programs, of which there are several in the United States, require an ultrasound examination and amniocentesis.[47] The prenatal diagnosis of these and many other anomalies is not easy. False negatives are common, as are false positives. Even with a detailed examination, the sacral portion of the fetal spine cannot be completely evaluated because of poorly defined landmarks in that area.

Gastroschisis, omphalocele, atresias of the small bowel, meconium ileus, and anal atresia have now been commonly diagnosed with ultrasound. Bilateral renal agenesis and hydronephrosis (unilateral or bilateral), osteogenesis imperfecta, short-limbed dwarfism, as well as a large number of rare and often subtle defects, have been reported as specifically diagnosed with ultrasound. Excellent reviews of this rapidly changing field are available which are beyond the scope of this chapter.[48-50]

The prenatal detection of some anomalies can be lifesaving, as, for example, the diaphragmatic hernia. But, unfortunately, ultrasound examination of *all* fetuses would be required to detect the majority of these cases before birth, a detection strategy that is currently not popular.

It cannot be overstated that detection of congenital anomalies is difficult and sometimes exquisitely subtle. The specialized examinations require a great deal of time, in many cases, and depend entirely on operator experience. In addition, even with a great deal of care and experience, *not all congenital anomalies can be diagnosed with diagnostic ultrasound*. The discrimination between normal and pathologic is a very subtle spectrum, which takes much experience to sort out.

This raises practical problems for clinical application of diagnostic ultrasound in obstetrics for two reasons: (1) the patient may have unrealistic expectations of her physician when this form of fetal observation is undertaken, and (2) failure to detect a major fetal abnormality may leave the inexperienced ultrasonographer at medicolegal jeopardy. In order to address these problems, a two-tiered approach to ultrasound prenatal diagnosis has been advocated by the Section of Obstetric and Gynecologic Ultrasound of the American Institute of Ultrasound in Medicine (AIUM). A stage I, or "standard obstetrical ultrasound examination," is meant specifically to obtain and document certain "baseline" fetal data, such as gestational age, estimated fetal size and weight, fetal number, presentation and life, placenta location, amniotic fluid volume estimate, and the appearance of certain major fetal anatomic landmarks, such as the head, limbs, kidneys and bladder, stomach, and heart. Any abnormality found at such an examination is an indication for a stage II ultrasound examination, that is now called a "second-opinion ultrasound consultation." This concept is still evolving, but has met with at least initial success in the obstetric office. In the future, when and if this two-tiered approach is coupled with routine ultrasound examination of all pregnancies at 16–20 weeks of age, it will be possible to test the hypothesis that such a strategy will improve the detection rate for major structural congenital anomalies, while providing both physicians and patients a large measure of protection and backup when abnormalities are thought to be present on ultrasound examination. At this time, however, there are no published, prospective, randomized studies to support this contention.

ANTEPARTUM ASSESSMENT OF FETAL WELL-BEING

In the past decade, perinatal mortality rates in the United States have declined markedly. The neonatal mortality rate has improved faster than the stillbirth rate, and antepartum and intrapartum assessment of fetal well-being has become an important part of high-risk obstetric management.

The biophysical profile was developed to assist perinatologists to discriminate between fetuses that are well adapted to their intrauterine environment and those that are in danger of intrauterine fetal demise that would do better being delivered.[51] The test consists of a set of five observations: (1) the first is based on the interpretation of a fetal-heart-rate-monitor tracing of the resting fetus [i.e., the Nonstress Test (NST)]; (2) the other four observations are of diagnostic ultrasound findings—the presence of fetal body movement (three in 30 minutes of observation), the presence of fetal chest wall movements (30 seconds worth of continuous breathing in 30 minutes), the observation of good fetal tone (one extension/flexion cycle of a fetal limb with rapid return to the flexed posture in 30 minutes), and the presence of a normal amount of amniotic fluid (i.e., greater than a 1-cm² "pocket" of fluid).

Each observed parameter receives a "planning score" of 2 or zero, depending on whether it meets the criteria outlined above or not. Ten is a "perfect" test result which is interpreted as reassuring. A zero, on the other hand, is the worst possible score, indicating a baby in extreme danger of dying in utero. It has been found that such observations are useful in the estimation of fetal well-being and in the reduction of perinatal mortality attributable to stillbirth in a high-risk obstetrical population. Furthermore, such a testing scheme can be used to identify "false-positive" results from the NST and/or Contraction Stress Test (CST), thus avoiding needless emergency intervention for a fetus in good condition in some circumstances.[52-54] This testing strategy is very much in the realm of clinical investigation. Only a few thousand patient tests and outcome have as yet been reported.

Such testing is required many times in the last few weeks of pregnancy. In some specific high-risk pregnancy situations, such testing may begin as early as 28 weeks and be carried out two or more times per week until delivery. From the biological-effects epidemiologic viewpoint, this will make the identification of any subtle biological effects of ultrasound very difficult, since the reasons for the multiple scans may be problems which will interfere with normal pregnancy outcome to a significant degree. Such babies are likely to exhibit a higher statistical frequency of low birth weight, prematurity, IUGR, and poor developmental performance across a broad spectrum of problems. At the same time, given the accepted efficacy of ultrasound use for the detection of fetal structural and functional abnormalities, the performance of prospective, randomized, blinded, controlled studies, to discern adverse or beneficial biological effects of diagnostic ultrasound on the human fetus, would almost certainly be unethical.

CONCLUDING REMARKS

There are no known or understood "side effects" from the use of diagnostic ultrasound on the human pregnant woman or fetus.[55] Except for supine hypotension, which can occur during the examination (from the weight of the uterus on the aorta and inferior vena cava as the woman lies on her back), no adverse patient reactions have ever been noted. This problem can be alleviated with the patient in a left tilt or in the left lateral recumbent position during the examination. The AIUM Clinical Safety Statement[56] (last revision, October 1983) represents that organization's official position regarding use of diagnostic ultrasound on patients.

> Diagnostic ultrasound has been in use for over 25 years. Given its known benefits and recognized efficacy for medical diagnosis, including use during human pregnancy, the American Institute of Ultrasound in Medicine herein addresses the clinical safety of such use:
> No confirmed biological effects on patients or instrument operators caused by exposure at intensities typical of present diagnostic ultrasound instruments have ever been reported. Although the possibility exists that such biological effects may be identified in the future, current data indicate that the benefits to patients of the prudent use of diagnostic ultrasound outweigh the risks, if any, that may be present.

The clinician will, in the future, benefit from electronic advances in diagnostic ultrasound image processing, the influence of computer and telecommunications technology, and from increased understanding of fetal pathophysiology in the presence of a seemingly ever-increasing diversity of abnormal conditions that are newly approachable in utero. Diagnostic ultrasound will always remain most useful as a confirmatory technology, used to provide adjunctive information to be integrated into the total patient data base of each women. All of those who perform and interpret diagnostic ultrasound information would do well to perform such interpretations with caution and specific attention to all the clinical information available for each patient. If that attitude is maintained and each practitioner seeks adequate training while utilizing consultants whenever uncertainty about ultrasound findings exists, then diagnostic ultrasound will continue to develop as the premier diagnostic technique for the fetus, to the direct benefit of all of the mothers and their children and families.

REFERENCES

1. Campbell S: The assessment of fetal development by diagnostic ultrasound. Br Med J 2:730, 1974
2. Dewhurst DJ, Beazley JM, Campbell S: Assessment of fetal maturity and dysmaturity. Am J Obstet Gynecol 113:14, 1972
3. Zador IE, Hertz RH, Sokol RJ, et al: Sources of error in the estimation of fetal gestational age. Am J Obstet Gynecol 138:344, 1980
4. Andersen HF, Johnson TRB, Barclay ML, et al: Gestational age assessment. Am J Obstet Gynecol 139:173, 1981
5. Hertz RH, Sokol RJ, Knoke JD, et al: Clinical estimation of gestational age: rules for avoiding preterm delivery. Am J Obstet Gynecol 131:395, 1978
6. Beazley JM, Underhill RA: Fallacy of the fundal height. Br Med J 4:404, 1970
7. Dubowitz LMS, Dubowitz V, Goldberg C: Clinical assessment of gestational age in the newborn infant. J Pediatr 77:1, 1970
8. Latis GO, Simionato L, Ferraris G: Clinical assessment of gestational age in the newborn infant: comparison of two methods. Early Hum Dev 5:29, 1980
9. Ounsted MK, Chalmers CA, Yudkin PL: Clinical assessment of gestational age at birth: the effects of sex, birthweight, and weight for length of gestation. Early Hum Dev 211:73, 1978
10. Jimenez JM, Tyson JE, Reisch JS: Clinical measures of gestational age in normal pregnancies. Obstet Gynecol 61:438, 1983
11. Kopta MM, May RR, Crane JP: A comparison of the reliability of the estimated date of confinement predicted by crown-rump length and biparietal diameter. Am J Obstet Gynecol 145:562, 1983
12. Aantaa K, Korrs M: Growth of the fetal biparietal diameter in different types of pregnancies. Radiology 137:167, 1980
13. Johnson ML, Dunne MC, Mack LA, et al: Evaluation of fetal intracranial anatomy by static and real time ultrasound. J Clin Ultrasound 8:311, 1980
14. Shepard M, Filly RA: A standardized plane for biparietal diameter measurement. J Ultrasound Med 1:145, 1982
15. Hadlock FP, Deter RL, Harrist RB, et al: Fetal biparietal diameter: rational choice of plane of section for sonographic measurement. Am J Roentgenol 138:871, 1982
16. Hadlock FP, Deter RL, Harrist RB, et al: Fetal biparietal diameter: a critical re-evaluation of the relation to menstrual age by means of real-time ultrasound. J Ultrasound Med 1:97, 1982
17. Kurtz AB, Wapner RJ, Kurtz RJ, et al: Analysis of biparietal diameter as an accurate indicator of gestational age. J Clin Ultrasound 8:319, 1980

18. Wiener SN, Flynn MJ, Kennedy AW, Bonk F: A composite curve of ultrasonic biparietal diameters for estimating gestational age. Radiology, 122:suppl. 2, 781, 1977

19. Sabbagha RE, Hughey M: Standardization of sonar cephalometry and gestational age. Obstet Gynecol 52:402, 1978

20. Sabbagha RE, Turner JH, Rockette H, et al: Sonar BPD and fetal age. Obstet Gynecol 43:7, 1974

21. Hohler CW, Quetel TA: Fetal femur length: Equations for computer calculation of gestational age from ultrasound measurements. Am J Obstet Gynecol 143:479, 1982

22. Hadlock FP, Deter RL, Harrist RB, et al: Fetal head circumference. Relation to menstrual age. Am J Roentgenol 138:649, 1982

23. Hadlock FP, Deter RL, Harrist RB, Park SK: Fetal abdominal circumference as a predictor of menstrual age. Am J Roentgenol 139:367, 1982

24. Deter RL, Harrist RB, Hadlock FP, et al: Longitudinal studies of fetal growth with dynamic image ultrasonography. Am J Obstet Gynecol 143:545, 1982

25. Tamura RK, Sabbagha RE: Percentile ranks of sonar fetal abdominal circumference measurements: Am J Obstet Gynecol 138:475, 1980

26. O'Brien GD, Queenan JT: Growth of the ultrasound fetal femur length during normal pregnancy. Am J Obstet Gynecol 141:833, 1981

27. Koops BL, Morgan LJ, Battaglia FC: Neonatal mortality risk in relation to birthweight and gestational age: update. J Pediatr 101:969, 1982

28. Starfield B, Shapiro S, McCormick M, Bross D: Mortality and morbidity in infants with intrauterine growth retardation. J Pediatr 101:978, 1982

29. Jones MD, Battaglia FC: Intrauterine growth retardation. Am J Obstet Gynecol 127:540, 1977

30. Bard H: Neonatal problems of infants with intrauterine growth retardation. J Reprod Med 21:359, 1978

31. Deter RL, Harrist RB, Hadlock FP, et al: The use of ultrasound in the detection of intrauterine growth retardation—a review. J Clin Ultrasound 10:9, 1982

32. Deter RL, Hadlock FP, Harrist RB, et al: Evaluation of three methods for obtaining fetal weight estimates using dynamic image ultrasound. J Clin Ultrasound 9:421, 1981

33. Shepard MJ, Richards VA, Berkowitz RL, et al: An evaluation of two equations for predicting fetal weight by ultrasound. Am J Obstet Gynecol 142:47, 1982

34. Deter RL, Hadlock FP, Harrist RB, et al: Fetal head and abdominal circumference. I. Evaluation of measurement errors. J Clin Ultrasound 10:357, 1982

35. Queenan JT, Kubarych SF, Cook LN, et al: Diagnostic ultrasound for detection of intrauterine growth retardation. Am J Obstet Gynecol 124:865, 1976

36. Hohler CW, Lea J, Collins H: Screening for intrauterine growth retardation using the ultrasound biparietal diameter. J Clin Ultrasound 4:187, 1977

37. Crane JP, Lopta MM, Welt DI, Sauvage JP: Abnormal fetal growth patterns: ultrasonic diagnosis and management. Obstet Gynecol 50:205, 1977

38. Campbell S, Thoms A: Ultrasound measurement of the fetal head to abdomen circumference ratio in the assessment of growth retardation. Br J Obstet Gynecol 84:165, 1977

39. Crane JP, Kopta MM: Prediction of intrauterine growth retardation via ultrasonically measured head/abdominal circumference ratios. Obstet Gynecol 54:497, 1979

40. Elliott JP, Garite TJ, Freeman RK, et al: Ultrasonic prediction of macrosomia in diabetic patients. Obstet Gynecol 60:159, 1982

41. Lubchenco LO, Hansman C, Dressler M, Boyd E: Intrauterine growth as estimated from liveborn birthweight data at 24 to 42 weeks of gestation. Pediatrics 32:793, 1963

42. Usher R, McLean F: Intrauterine growth of liveborn Caucasian infants at sea level: standards obtained from measurements in 7 dimensions of infants born between 25 and 44 weeks of gestation. Pediatrics 74:901, 1969

43. Brenner WE, Edelman DA, Hendricks CH: A standard fetal growth for the United States of America. Am J Obstet Gynecol 126:555, 1976

44. Miller HC, Hassanein K: Diagnosis of impaired fetal growth in newborn infants. Pediatrics 48:511, 1971

45. Daikoku NH, Johnson JWC, Graf C, et al: Patterns of intrauterine growth retardation. Obstet Gynecol 54:211, 1979

46. Queenan JT, Gadow EC: Amniography for detection of congenital malformations. Obstet Gynecol 36:648, 1970

47. Macri JN, Weiss RR: Prenatal serum alpha-fetoprotein screening for neural tube defects. Obstet Gynecol 59:633, 1982

48. Dunne MG, Johnson ML: The ultrasonic demonstration of fetal abnormalities in utero. J Reprod Med 23:195, 1979

49. Hadlock FP, Deter RL, Carpenter R, et al: Review. Sonography of fetal urinary tract anomalies. Am J Roentgenol 137:261, 1981

50. Hobbins JC, Grannum PAT, Berkowitz RL, et al: Ultrasound in the diagnosis of congenital anomalies. Am J Obstet Gynecol 134:331, 1979

51. Manning FA, Platt LD, Sipos L: Antepartum fetal evaluation: development of a fetal biophysical profile. Am J Obstet Gynecol 136:787, 1980

52. Schifrin BS, Guntes V, Gergely RC, et al: The role of real-time scanning in antenatal fetal surveillance. Am J Obstet Gynecol 140:525, 1981

53. Manning FA, Morrison I, Lange IR, et al: Antepartum determination of fetal health: composite biophysical profile scoring. Clin Perinatol 9:285, 1982

54. Platt LD, Eglinton GS, Sipos L, et al: Further experience with the fetal biophysical profile. Obstet Gynecol 61:480, 1983

55. Hohler CW: Ultrasound bioeffects for the perinatologist. Chapter 71. In Sciarra J (ed): Gynecology and Obstetrics. Vol. 3. Harper and Row, New York, 1984

56. AIUM Bioeffects Committee: Safety considerations for diagnostic ultrasound, p. 3. American Institute of Ultrasound in Medicine. Bethesda, Md., 1984

10 Epidemiology and Human Exposure

MARVIN C. ZISKIN

No matter how many laboratory experiments show a lack of effect from diagnostic ultrasound, it will always be necessary to study directly its effect in human populations before any definitive statement regarding risk can be made. As we have learned from our experiences with drug toxicity, drugs deemed "safe" following extensive laboratory experimentation have been found later to produce adverse effects when administered to large numbers of patients. Furthermore, the unexpected damage may be quite serious and still may not become apparent until many years following the actual exposure. It took approximately 20 years for vaginal cancer to show up in daughters of women who had taken diethylstibestrol (DES) during pregnancy. It was also approximately 20 years before thyroid cancer became evident in indviduals who as children had been exposed to radiation therapy of their thymus glands. These delayed effects illustrate the need for long-term as well as short-term studies of exposure of human populations to external agents such as ultrasound.

CLINICAL SURVEYS

The study of the effects of ultrasonic exposure on human populations is in the province of epidemiology. Perhaps the simplest and most rudimentary form of epidemiologic study is the clinical survey, of which several have been performed. These surveys dealt with examinations of patients in which commercial instruments were used; acoustic output data were not specified.

In 1972, Ziskin[1] reported on an international survey of clinical users of diagnostic ultrasound. He reported that no adverse effects attributed to examination by ultrasound had been identified by any of the 68 respondents to the survey in over 121,000 patient examinations. The report represented a combined total of 292 institute-years of experience in the clinical use of diagnostic ultrasound. A national survey of clinical users was carried out in 1980 by the Environmental Health Directorate of Canada.[2] From the replies it was estimated that 340,000 patients were examined with diagnostic ultrasound in 1977 for a total of 1.2 million examinations. Only one adverse effect on a patient was reported by the 111 respondents, and its nature was not identified. Statistical considerations indicate that these large surveys give strong evidence against ultrasound producing obvious abnormalities which are evident soon after the exposure and which in the absence of any exposure are rare. However, even such large surveys are not well suited for detecting small changes in the rate of more common occurrences.

While it is reassuring that these two surveys of clinical users of ultrasound found no clear example of an adverse effect, it must be pointed out that it is not known how diligently these users were looking for adverse effects or what kinds of effects they were looking for. Perhaps the fairest statement to be made is that based on 461,000 patient examinations, 179 clinical users overwhelmingly believed that their experiences with ultrasound had been safe.

In 1974, Ford[3] examined the brains at autopsy of 24 neurologic and neurosurgical patients who had multiple ultrasonic pulse-echo examinations at up to 120 days prior to death. He could not detect any changes attributable to the ultrasound.

In 1967, Kohorn et al.[4] examined 20 normal babies during the first 3 days of life. The output from a diagnostic pulse-echo instrument was applied to the head of each new-born baby for a 10 minute exposure. No alterations in electroencephalogram (EEG) tracings were detected following the ultrasound exposure.

Timmermans,[5] in 1973, exposed the urologic tract of 300 patients to the output of a 2.25-MHz pulsed diagnostic instrument and found no detectable disorders.

STUDIES OF FETAL EXPOSURE

A number of attempts has been made to determine whether diagnostic ultrasound effects the human fetus. A good review has been completed by Scheidt and Lundin.[6] Commercial equipment was used in applying the diagnostic ultrasound for all of the investigations reviewed here. Unfortunately, acoustic output data were usually not stated.

The largest completed study considered in the above-mentioned review was conducted by Hellman et al.[7] It consisted of a retrospective, but not case-controlled, study of 1,114 apparently normal pregnant women examined by ultrasound in the United States, Sweden, and Scotland. A 2.7 percent incidence of congenital abnormalities was found by newborn physical examination in this group, as compared with a figure of 4.8 percent reported in a separate and unmatched survey of women who had not been examined with ultrasound. Hellman et al. concluded that neither the frequency of the ultrasound examination nor the time of the first examination seems to effect adversely the overall incidence of fetal abnormality and abortion.

It is interesting to note that, based on a sample size of 1,114 patients, the observed decrease in the incidence of fetal abnormalities from 4.8 to 2.7 percent is statistically significant ($p < 0.01$). It is not known how to interpret this finding, since the exposed and unexposed groups were not matched. For example, it is possible that information derived from ultrasound examinations was used as an indicator for therapeutic abortions; if so, fewer abnormalities would have been expected among full-term births. In any event, this finding vividly points out the caution that must be exercised in interpreting the results of an epidemiologic study. This is especially true when the study has inadequately matched controls. Ideally, subjects should be randomly selected to experimental and control groups to avoid inadvertent biases in the analysis.

Other studies have been performed which show no significant change produced by diagnostic ultrasound. Bernstein[8] exposed 720 fetuses in utero to 6-MHz continuous-wave (CW) Doppler ultrasound at an intensity (I_t: spatial-average temporal-average intensity measured at the transducer face; see Chapter 2) of 20–30 mW/cm². He was unable to detect any difference in the incidence of obstetric complications resulting from exposure to ultrasound.

Scheidt et al.[9] studied 1907 infants with respect to 123 variables including those concerned with pregnancy, delivery, and the neonatal period. Intensity data for the ultrasound equipment were apparently not available. While 297 infants were exposed to ultrasound in utero and had amniocentesis, 661 had amniocentesis only, and 949 had neither. Clinical follow-up at 1 year of age included a history, physical examination, and the Denver Development Screening Test. There were more grasp and tonic neck reflex abnormalities in the group with both ultrasound and amniocentesis than in the group with neither, but no such difference existed between the group with both ultrasound and amniocentesis and the group with amniocentesis alone. There were no other statistically significant findings.

In two separate reports dealing with the same study, Falus et al.[10] and Koranyi et al.[11] examined 171 children aged 6 months to 3 years who had been exposed to ultrasound in utero. Physical examinations and histories led the investigators to conclude that bodily and mental development was average or better. Karyotype analysis of 10 exposed children and 10 control children failed to reveal any differences.

Other studies also producing negative results were performed by Serr et al.[12] on 150 exposed fetuses, by Watts and Steward[13] on 10 mothers at term, by Ikeuchi et al.[14] on 98 first-trimester fetuses, and by Abdulla et al.[15] on 35 second-trimester fetuses.

Using data from a larger long-term study of children exposed to ultrasound in utero, Moore et al.[16] analyzed a subset of previously accumulated records of 2,135 single births (half of them exposed) for the possibility of a reduction in birth weight due to the ultrasound. Upon finding a crude association which was statistically significant ($p < 0.01$), they limited their attention to 527 single births for more detailed analysis in which they adjusted for demographic characteristics, previous pregnancy history, and some events during pregnancy. Then, with these adjustments, they were still able to show a small but statistically significant ($p < 0.05$) decrease in the mean birth weight of the exposed infants.

Analyzing a different subset of this same data base, Stark et al.[17] found no relationship between ultrasound exposure and birthweight. In addition to birth weight, a number of physical, developmental, neurological, and psychological measurements were performed at birth and at age 7–12 years. No significant differences between the exposed and unexposed children were observed. However, there was a tendency (not statistically significant unless data from all three hospitals involved in the study were pooled) for higher incidence of dyslexia in the ultrasound-exposed children at 7–12 years.

Although refuted by Stark et al.,[17] the report by Moore et al.[16] is important because of the positive findings. However, it must be noted that the data in both of these reports were analyzed several years after they had been collected and that the reasons for which pregnant women did or did not receive the ultrasound are not known. The possibility that a problem pregnancy would have been more likely to receive the ultrasound than a normal one cannot be discounted even with the adjustments made in the analysis. It should also be noted that adjustments for smoking or for the physical sizes of the parents were not included in the analysis. All these factors introduce possible biases and weaken the conclusions reached.

The largest study is currently under way in Canada under the direction of E.A. Lyons.[18] Ten thousand pregnant women who were exposed to ultrasound will be identified and matched with 500 controls. Data extracted from medical records and long-term follow-up evaluations of the offspring will be studied. In a preliminary report, Lyons and Coggrave-Toms[19] followed 2,428 children. They reported no evidence for increased incidence of congenital malformations, chromosome abnormalities, neoplasms, speech or hearing disorders, or developmental problems.

A number of studies has been made to determine whether chromosome damage has occurred in the mother and/or fetus following ultrasound examinations. Although the results were not statistically significant, Serr et al.[12] suggested that damage to the chromosomes of fetal cells obtained by amniocentesis may have occurred following a 10-hour exposure to 6-MHz ultrasound of intensity 22 mW/cm^2 (probably I_t). This suggestion is in contrast to Ikeuchi et al.[14] who found no chromosome damage in 98 first-trimester fetuses exposed for 5 minutes to 20-MHz CW ultrasound at 20 mW/cm^2 (probably I_t). Also, Abdulla et al.[15] did not find any increase in chromosome abnormalities in maternal or fetal lymphocytes following exposure to 1.5-MHz pulsed ultrasound or to 2-MHz CW ultrasound. Intensities, cited as temporal and spatial averages measured 10 cm from the transducer were 0.8 mW/cm^2 for the pulsed and either 0.8 mW/cm^2 or 22 mW/cm^2 for the CW ultrasound.

In addition to fetal exposures, a recent report, unconfirmed, suggests that premature ovulation may occur following the use of certain ovulation-induction medications when ultrasonic scanning (intensities unspecified) is used in the late follicular phase.[20]

EFFECT ON FETAL ACTIVITY

In 1975, David et al.[21] reported a 90 percent increase in fetal activity during a 15-minute exposure of CW Doppler ultrasound following a 15-minute control period. This was considered to be of general medical interest and not an indication of harmful effect. Fetal activity was determined by the number of times a mother reported the subjective sensation of fetal movement. This study, performed on 36 mothers, had a number of serious design flaws, such as the subjective nature of test variable and the sequence in which the test period always followed the control period.

Another study of fetal activity was reported in 1979 by Powell-Phillips and Towell.[22] They used an objective strain gauge measurement for defining fetal movement. They were unable to show any increase in fetal activity during ultrasound exposure, thus shedding doubt on the previous study. The major limitation of the latter study was that only 25 patients were evaluated.

Hertz et al.[23] also studied the possibility of fetal activity being increased during CW ultrasonic examination. They also obtained negative results. However, their study was even smaller, with only 13 patients.

STATISTICAL CONSIDERATIONS

If the biological effects of diagnostic ultrasound exposure were obvious and frequent, there might not be a need for statistics to assess the risk. However, adverse effects, if any at all, are certainly not obvious and statistical methods will be required for their detection.

The ability to detect an adverse effect depends on a number of factors. Perhaps the three most important are (1) the visibility or conspicuousness of the effect if it does occur; (2) whether the effect constitutes a new event or, instead, an increase in the incidence of naturally occurring event, and; (3) the magnitude of the increase in incidence of a naturally occurring event.

In general, the smaller and less obvious the effect, the more difficult it is to be detected and the larger the sample size must be in order for a study to prove its existence.

Table 10.1 shows the minimum number of subjects required in a study in order to conclude that an observed increase in incidence is statistically significant. For example, suppose that a study has been performed to determine whether ultrasound if applied during pregnancy causes congenital abnormalities. The investigators report that 6 percent of the infants exposed in utero had congenital abnormalities as compared to a 5 percent natural (unexposed) incidence rate. The one-percentage-point increase could have come about in one of two ways: (1) ultrasound has no effect and the increase occurred by pure chance, or (2) the ultrasound did in fact cause an increase in the number of congenital abnormalities. Reference to Table 10.1 shows that in order for an observed one-percentage-point increase above 5 percent to be statistically significant, the minimum sample size would have to be 1,294.

It is customary to use a 5 percent significance level in deciding which of these two alternatives is correct. The underlying statistical reasoning is as follows:

Assume ultrasound has no effect. Were we able to observe the universe of all infants, we would obtain the true natural incidence (5 percent in the present

TABLE 10.1 Minimum sample size required to detect adverse effect of ultrasound[a]

Observed Increase in Incidence Following Ultrasound (in Percent-Point Difference)	Naturally Occurring Incidence of Event			
	5%	10%	20%	50%
10	13	25	69	69
5	52	99	174	273
2	324	613	1,089	1,702
1	1,294	2,451	4,356	6,807
0.5	5,200	9,801	17,400	27,225
0.1	129,400	245,100	435,600	680,700

[a] The values in this table are based on the commonly accepted 5% significant level. The statistical power is 0.5.

example). However, any given study involves only a sample of infants and the measured incidence may be higher or lower than the true incidence. The probability of the size of any deviation can readily be determined. Large deviations are less likely than small deviations. If a deviation as large as the observed deviation (one percentage point in the present example) is to be expected less than 5 percent of the time, we conclude that the sample is truly different from the universe of unexposed infants. Then, if exposure to ultrasound was the only difference between these groups, we would mistakenly conclude that ultrasound caused the effect.

The use of the 5 percent significance level is quite reasonable in that it will permit us to make the right decision 95 percent of the time. Conversely, however, we must forget that we will be wrong 5 percent of the time. This is one of the reasons why different studies addressing the same question will produce contradictory results. It is also important to note that even if diagnostic ultrasound produces no adverse effects at all, we should expect that 5 out of every 100 studies will report some positive finding.

If the hypothesized increase in incidence had been 0.5 percent instead of 1 percent (that is, the observed incidence was 5.5 percent instead of 6 percent) the sample size would have had to be quadrupled in order to establish the presence of a true effect. In this case the sample size would have had to be at least 5,200.

The above considerations were based on a number of assumptions, which if not correct would require even larger sample sizes. For example, it was assumed that the naturally occurring incidence was known. If this is not true then an equally large control group would also be required.

It is also possible to determine for a given sample size, how large a detected increase in incidence must be in order to be statistically significant. For example, in the study by Bernstein[8] of 720 pregnancies, the U.S. Navy-wide incidence of prematurity was 7.9 percent. For any observed increase to be statistically significant, the observed incidence would have had to exceed 9.5 percent (a relative increase of over 20 percent). This points out that even what might appear as a reasonably large study is quite limited in its ability to detect small changes in incidence, if the naturally occurring frequency is appreciable in the general population.

In planning a new study, one must also be concerned about the probability that the proposed study will actually be able to detect a true effect. This is referred to as the statistical power of the study. In the preceding example, the statistical power would have been only 50 percent. This means that even with the large sample sizes mentioned, a true effect would not be found 50 percent of the time. In order to obtain an 80 percent probability of detecting a true effect, the sample size would need to be more than doubled over those previously determined.

The purpose of this discussion has been to demonstrate (1) the importance of considering the statistical power of a study and (2) the very large sample sizes required to achieve any reasonable likelihood of detecting a small increase in incidence of a naturally occurring event.

THE VALUE OF NEGATIVE SURVEYS

A number of clinical surveys described in this chapter have reported an absence of any adverse effects due to ultrasound. Although described as negative, these surveys do provide information relative to risk.

Statistical theory permits us to quantitate the significance of nonobservance of adverse effects, provided that they can be detected if they occur. That is, based on the number of patient examination studies, we can state that the probability of such an effect is less than some amount (with 95 percent confidence). The exact relationship is given by

$$p \leq 1 - (0.05)^{1/N}$$

where p is the probability of the effect under consideration and N is the number of patient examinations studied.

For example, suppose that there have been no cases of a missing right thumb in 10,000 live births of infants who received ultrasound in utero. In this case,

$$p \leq 1 - (0.05)^{1/10,000} = 0.0003$$

Thus, we can be 95 percent confident that the true occurrence of this effect is less than 0.030 percent. If we had wished to be more conservative and had demanded to be 99 percent confident, 0.01 would have been substituted for 0.05 in the above equation, and we would have obtained a maximum occurrence rate of 0.046 percent.

Consider the survey by Ziskin of 121,000 patient examinations in which no adverse effects were reported. One can utilize the above equation to provide an upper limit to the probability of occurrence for any gross effect which practically never occurs in the absence of ultrasound and hence would have been seen and reported had it occurred:

$$p \leq 1 - (0.05)^{1/121,000} = 0.000025$$

Thus if the unusual event under consideration occurs at all, its rate of occurrence must be very low, specifically less than 25 in one million examinations. Analysis of findings from the survey carried out by the Canadian Environmental Health Directorate leads to similar conclusions.

It is clear that the absence of positive findings in such a survey provides useful information on rare events. However, events would have to be obvious to the observers and the sample size would have to be large in order for the results to be meaningful. For example, consider the study by Kohorn et al.[4] who found no EEG tracing alterations in 20 infants. Applying the same equation we see that the true incidence of EEG alterations could have been as high as 14 percent of all infants without being detected.

While large clinical surveys are valuable in testing for unusual events, they are not sensitive instruments for dealing with more common ones. For example, an obstetrician, Dr. A, would respond to the questionnaire by considering his records, which include observations of anomalies in infants, some of whom were exposed to diagnostic ultrasound prenatally, and some not. Dr. A would necessarily report "No adverse effects attributed to ultrasound" even though anomalies were observed among the exposed group, unless their number significantly exceeds the number expected in an equal population of unexposed infants. Judgments on "significance" are dependent on a number of factors, such as those discussed above, and a negative reply to a clinical survey can represent a range of possibilities.

CONCLUDING REMARKS

It appears from findings reviewed in this chapter that epidemiological studies and surveys of clinical experience have yielded no firm evidence of any adverse effects from diagnostic ultrasound, in spite of large clinical usage. This apparent safety is of paramount importance to the physician. While recognizing the limitations of clinical trials, these still represent to the physician the most sensitive and ultimate tests of any drug or agent. In the physician's experience, even when all laboratory tests have been free of adverse effects, unexpected untoward reactions will frequently be seen when any given agent is administered to a large number of patients.

The inability to find convincing proof of an effect, either from epidemiology or from the physician's experience, does not preclude the possibility of it happening. Statistical reasoning shows that even with large population studies, it is difficult to identify a small increase in rate of a commonly occurring event, even if each event is easily seen. Also subtle effects (such as minor chemical changes and minor behavioral changes), long-term delayed effects, and certain genetic effects could easily escape detection.

REFERENCES

1. Ziskin MC: Survey of patient exposure to diagnostic ultrasound. p. 203. In Reid JM, Sikov MR (eds): Interaction of Ultrasound and Biological Tissues. Department of Health, Education and Welfare Publication (FDA) 78–8008. Government Printing Office, Washington, DC, 1972

2. Environmental Health Directorate: Safety Code 23 Guidelines for the Safe Use of Ultrasound. Part I. Medical and Paramedical Applications, Report 8-EDH-59. Environmental Health Directorate, Health Protection Branch, Ottawa, Canada, 1981

3. Ford RM: Clinical-pathological studies on brain tissue response to ultrasonic radiation: preliminary results. p. 85. In de Vlieger M, White DN, and McCready VR (eds): Ultrasonics in Medicine. Excerpta Medica, Amsterdam, 1974

4. Kohorn ET, Pritchard JW, Hobbins JC: The safety of clinical ultrasonic examination. Obstet Gynecol 29:272, 1967

5. Timmermans L: Les ultrasons dans le diagnostic des maladies des reins de la prostate. Acta Urol Belg 41:337, 1973

6. Scheidt PC, Lundin FE: Investigations for effects of intrauterine ultrasound in humans. p. 19. In Hazzard DG, Litz, ML (eds): Symposium on Biological Effects and Characterizations of Ultrasound Sources. Department of Health, Education and Welfare Publication (FDA) 78–8048. Government Printing Office, Washington, DC, 1972

7. Hellman LM, Duffus GM, Ronald I, Sunden B: Safety of diagnostic ultrasound in obstetrics. Lancet 1:1133, 1970

8. Bernstein RL: Safety studies with ultrasonic Doppler technique: a clinical follow-up of patients and tissue culture study. Obstet Gynecol 34:707, 1969

9. Scheidt PC, Stanley F, Bryla DA: One year follow-up of infants exposed to ultrasound in utero. Am J Obstet Gynecol 131:743, 1978

10. Falus M, Koranyi G, Sobel M, et al.: Follow-up studies on infants examined by ultrasound during the fetal age. Orv Hetilao 13:2119, 1972

11. Koranyi G, Falus M, Sobel M, et al.: Follow-up examination of children exposed to ultrasound in utero. Arch Otolaryngol 86:83, 1972

12. Serr DM, Padeh B, Zakat H, et al: Studies on the effect of ultrasonic waves on the fetus. p. 302. In Huntington PJ, Beard RW, Hutton EE, et al (eds): Proceedings Second European Congress on Perinatal Medicine. London, 1971

13. Watts PL, Stewart CR: The effect of fetal heart monitoring by ultrasound on maternal and fetal chromosomes. J Obstet Gynaecol Br Commonw 72:715, 1972

14. Ikeuchi T, Sasaki M, Oshimura M, et al: Ultrasound and embryonic chromosomes. Br Med J 1:112, 1973

15. Abdulla U, Dewhurst CJ, Campbell C, et al: Effect of diagnostic ultrasound on maternal and fetal chromosomes. Lancet 2:829, 1971

16. Moore RM, Jr, Barrick KM, Hamilton TM: Effect of sonic radiation on growth and development. In Proceedings Meeting of the Society for Epidemiologic Research, Cincinnati, OH, June 16–18, 1982

17. Stark CR, Orleans M, Havercamp AD, Murphy J: Short- and long-term risks after exposure to diagnostic ultrasound in utero. Obstet Gynecol 63:194, 1984

18. Lyons EA, Coggrave M, Brown RE: Follow-up study in children exposed to ultrasound in utero-analysis of height and weight in the first six years of life. p. 49. In Proceedings 25th Annual Meeting of American Institute of Ultrasound in Medicine, New Orleans, LA, September 15–19, 1980

19. Lyons EA, Coggrave-Toms M: Long term follow-up study of children exposed to ultrasound in utero. p. 112. In Proceedings 24th Annual Meeting of American Institute of Ultrasound in Medicine, Montreal, Canada, August 27–31, 1979

20. Testart J, Inserm U, Thebault A, et al: Premature ovulation after ovarian ultrasonography, Br J Obstet Gynaecol 89:694, 1982

21. David H, Weaver JB, Pearson JF (1975): Doppler ultrasound and fetal activity. Br Med J 2:62, 1975

22. Powell-Phillips WD, Towell ME: Doppler ultrasound and subjective assessment of fetal activity. Br Med J 2:101, 1979

23. Hertz RH, Timor-Tritsch I, Diercker LJ, et al: Continuous ultrasound and fetal movement. Am J Obstet Gynecol 135:152, 1979

11 Therapeutic Applications of Ultrasound

MARY DYSON

Ultrasound has been used as a therapeutic agent, mainly as a means of stimulating the repair of soft tissue injuries and relieving pain, for over 40 years. The types of injuries treated include damage to ligaments, joint capsules, tendons and muscles, inflammation of tendon sheaths, scar tissue tension and sensitivity, pressure sores and varicose ulcers, fasciitis, amputation neuromata and treatment soreness.[1] Some idea of the scale on which ultrasound is used as a therapeutic agent can be gathered from data in a recent publication based on a national survey by the Environmental Health Directorate of Canada (1980)[2] in which it was reported that in 1977 nearly 4,000,000 ultrasonic treatments were given in Canada alone, compared with approximately 1,200,000 examinations with diagnostic ultrasound. In the United Kingdom virtually all hospital physiotherapists have access to ultrasonic therapy machines, as do those associated with sports medicine. The widespread and apparently increasing use of ultrasound as a therapeutic agent is mainly due to its effectiveness and excellent safety record when used correctly. Incorrect usage at best reduces the beneficial effects of ultrasonic therapy and at worst can result in tissue damage. Correct usage can only be ensured if the therapist has access to reliable, accurately calibrated equipment, and has an adequate understanding both of the effects of ultrasound on the cells and tissues being treated and of the physical mechanisms by which these effects are produced.

ULTRASONIC THERAPY EQUIPMENT

An ultrasonic therapy machine of the kind currently available commercially consists of a high-frequency generator linked, typically, to a transducer housed in a submersible hand-held applicator. The transducer is usually a flat disc of piezoelectric ceramic material such as lead zirconate titanate. Although many machines operate at only one frequency, typically 1 MHz, the more versatile operate at a range of frequencies, for example, 0.75, 1.5, and 3 MHz. Some can produce only a continuous beam of ultrasound, while others allow the beam to be emitted in either continuous or pulsed mode. When available, the pulses are typically 1 msec or 2 msec long and are separated by spaces of 1, 2, or 8 msec duration. The effective radiating area of the transducer is generally about 5 cm², although there is a need for smaller transducers, housed in tapered applicators, to facilitate the treatment of smaller units of tissue and the application of ultrasound to irregular skin surfaces by direct contact. The power output of the machines can generally be varied, either continuously or discontinuously, to give spatial-average temporal-average intensities (I_t, as defined in Chapter 2) in the range of 0.1–3.0 W/cm². Most machines are equipped with timers and give an audible signal on completion of the set treatment time. An additional refinement on some machines is a warning light or an audible signal which operates if acoustic coupling to the target is inadequate.

METHOD OF APPLICATION OF ULTRASONIC THERAPY

Because ultrasound at megahertz frequencies is greatly attenuated by reflection at air-tissue boundaries, it has to be applied to the skin via a coupling agent which displaces the air. Sterile degassed water is an excellent coupling medium, and lesions on the extremities, for example, can be readily treated in a bath in which both the target and the applicator can be submerged. The bath should be lined with an ultrasound absorbing material such as rubber matting to minimize reflection at the interface between the water-filled container and the surrounding air. Where submersion of the affected region in water is inconvenient, an alternative method is to couple the applicator to the skin via a thin film of oil, acoustic coupling cream, or a water-based gel. These coupling agents have the advantage of lubricating the skin so that the applicator can be moved over it easily, as well as causing little attenuation of the ultrasound. If the surface to be treated is very irregular and cannot be readily submerged in water, a deformable water-filled latex cushion, coated with a thin film of one of the coupling agents listed above, can be placed in contact with the region to be treated and the ultrasound applied through it. Whatever the coupling medium selected, care must be taken to ensure that it remains air-free throughout the treatment period, thereby permitting uninterrupted ultrasound transmission into the patient.

Once the ultrasound has been successfully led into the skin from a flat disc transducer, it travels as an approximately cylindrical but gradually diverging beam through the various tissues of the body, being differentially attenuated by them. The ultrasonic intensity applied initially decreases exponentially with the distance traveled as a result of absorption and scattering. Absorption results in heating, and varies according to the composition of the tissues in the path of the beam, those tissues with a high protein content absorbing ultrasound more readily than those with a high fat content. Highly collagenous tendons, joint capsules, and ligaments are thus heated more than, for example, the skin and subcutaneous adipose tissues covering them, when treated with therapeutic levels of ultrasound. Scattering is due to the heterogeneity of the tissues, for they contain and are separated by acoustic interfaces which reflect energy away from the main beam and thus make heating effects more diffuse. Both absorption and scattering increase with frequency, so the higher the frequency used the greater the attenuation. For practical purposes attenuation can be conveniently quantified in terms of *half-value thickness,* that is, the distance traveled by an ultrasonic beam before it is reduced to half its original value. In skin and loose connective tissue at 1 MHz the half-value thickness is approximately 40 mm, while at 2.5 MHz this is decreased to 16 mm. The half-life thickness for fat at 2.5 MHz is approximately 20 mm and that for bone is less than 1 mm; by contrast, the half-value thickness for blood at 2.5 MHz is over 65 mm. The amount of ultrasound reaching the site of a deeply situated lesion thus depends upon the frequency of the ultrasound used and the nature and thickness of the more superficially located tissues.

The target is also affected by tissues lying deep to it. If there is a significant change of acoustic impedance at their interfaces these will reflect much of the ultrasound which has traveled beyond the target. If, in addition to this, the applicator and the reflecting interface are stationary, standing waves may be produced, causing large local increases in intensity and in heating at half-wavelength intervals. The interfaces between soft tissue and bone, soft tissue and gases, and soft tissue and metal implants, all reflect ultrasound sufficiently to induce standing-wave production. To reduce the time of exposure of tissues to the localized high acoustic amplitudes induced by standing waves, for example, it is generally recommended that the applicator be moved in a regular and continuous fashion throughout the entire treatment period of from 5–10 minutes.

THERAPEUTIC EFFECTS OF ULTRASOUND

These can be classified into those where there is evidence that their primary cause is the increase in temperature induced by ultrasound, and those in which nonthermal mechanisms, such as acoustic streaming and/or stable cavitation play a significant role.

Thermally Induced Therapeutic Effects

For an effect induced by ultrasound to be attributable primarily to heating, it should be possible to duplicate it by nonacoustically produced heating, provided that the temperature history during heating and cooling duplicates the temperature history during ultrasonic irradiation.[3] Many of the therapeutic effects of ultrasound appear to fall into this category. They include increase in the extensibility of collagen-rich structures such as tendons and joint capsules, decrease in joint stiffness, reduction of pain, reduction of muscle spasms, and production of a mild inflammatory reaction including a marked increase in blood flow which may help in the resolution of chronic inflammatory processes.[4] Similar effects can be produced if the tissue temperature is raised by nonacoustic means to reach the range of 40–45°C. Temperatures below this range are ineffective, while temperatures above 45°C are potentially destructive. Furthermore, the temperature must remain within the range of 40–45°C for at least 5 minutes to produce the effects listed above.

The main advantage of using ultrasound rather than a nonacoustic method to raise the temperature locally is that ultrasound allows collagen-rich tissues to be heated preferentially. Scar tissue, joint capsules, and tendons lying deep within the body can therefore be heated to the therapeutically effective range without producing damaging temperature elevations in the skin and subcutaneous adipose tissue lying superficial to them. Other anatomic structures that can be heated preferentially with ultrasound include the periosteum, superficial cortical bone, joint menisci, fibrotic muscle, tendon sheaths, and the major nerve roots.[4] Recently it was also found that intermuscular interfaces could be heated selectively.[5] Another advantage is that since the depth of penetration is inversely related to frequency, the depth at which significant thermal effects occur can to some extent be controlled when ultrasound is used as the means of inducing a local rise in temperature. The temperature distribution induced by ultrasound in human tissues when it is used at therapeutic levels is far from uniform, however, and is further complicated by thermal diffusion and temperature changes induced by the flow of blood through the irradiated tissues.

Whenever ultrasound is used as a means of heating, it should be appreciated that nonthermal changes can occur simultaneously with increase in temperature, and can interact, either constructively or destructively, with thermally induced effects. The results of raising tissue temperature locally by irradiation with therapeutic ultrasound are therefore not necessarily the same as raising it to the same extent by nonacoustic means.

Nonthermally Induced Therapeutic Effects

The use of ultrasound at levels below those inducing the physiologically significant temperature increases described above can be of therapeutic advantage in a variety of ways in the treatment of injured tissues. Although some local increase in tissue temperature does occur and may be involved in the beneficial results obtained, it is now widely accepted that the nonthermal events which accompany this play a greater role in their production. In some instances there is experimental evidence for this[6-8] while in others it can be inferred from the treatment parameters used.

Examples of therapeutically significant effects of ultrasound thought to have a primarily nonthermal causation include the stimulation of tissue regeneration,[6] soft tissue repair,[7, 9] blood flow in chronically ischemic tissues,[8] protein synthesis,[10] bone repair,[11] induction of repair of ununited bone fractures (Duarte LR: personal communication), the relief of postherpetic pain (Oakley EM: personal communication), and phonophoresis.[12] Other therapeutic applications of ultrasound which fall into this category have been described by Summer and Patrick.[13]

Nonthermally induced therapeutic effects can be obtained by using lower intensities (I_t) than those necessary to ensure physiologically significant levels of heating. Instead of intensities (I_t) of 0.5–3.0 W/cm², I_t levels of 0.1 W/cm² and 0.2 W/cm² are typically employed. Although these low levels can be achieved in continuous mode, they are most commonly achieved by using the pulsed mode with SATP intensities in the range of 0.5–1.0 W/cm² and a duty cycle of about 0.2.

NONTHERMAL MECHANISMS INVOLVED IN THE PRODUCTION OF THERAPEUTIC EFFECTS

The physical mechanisms currently believed to be involved in ultrasonic therapy at levels below those necessary to produce physiologically significant heating include acoustic streaming and cavitation.[14, 15] See Chapter 3.

Acoustic streaming is the unidirectional movement of fluid in an ultrasonic pressure field. Connective tissue fibers and the plasma membranes of immobile cells form boundaries in the ultrasonic pressure field, and at these boundaries high velocity gradients develop. Similar effects occur at the surface of any gas bubbles present in the field. Acoustic streaming subjects the boundaries to considerable shear stress. If the boundary is the membrane of a cell the changes induced in it can affect aspects of the cell's behavior which can produce therapeutically significant effects (see below). When the geometrical scale of acoustic streaming is sufficiently small (microscopically detectable) it is often referred to as *microstreaming.*[16]

Cavitation has been defined as any observable activity involving a bubble or a population of bubbles stimulated into motion by an acoustic field.[17] It concentrates acoustic energy in localized high stresses, elevated temperatures, and/or fluid velocities, any of which can affect the activities of cells exposed to them. The type of cavitation likely to be involved in the production of therapeutically useful effects is the stable variety in which gas bubbles a few microns in size oscillate in a regular fashion for many acoustic cycles. The enhanced microstreaming induced around them may be responsible, at least in part, for changes which have been observed in the permeability of the cell membrane to ions such as sodium[18] and calcium[19] after treatment with therapeutic levels of ultrasound.

Changes in permeability to sodium ions may be responsible for the altered electrical activity which has been observed in nerve[20, 21] and muscle[22] following treatment with therapeutic levels of ultrasound; the possibility that such alterations may be involved in the relief of pain and the reduction of muscle spasm reputedly produced by certain methods of ultrasonic therapy treatment (see above) remains to be investigated. Changes in permeability to calcium ions may have dramatic effects on cell behavior. Calcium ion fluxes act as chemical signals, "second messengers" which, in response to membrane changes, control the enzymatic machinery of the cell, and stimulate, for example, controlled increase in the synthesis of specific proteins and their secretion. These latter effects are clearly of important value therapeutically in the recovery of cells and tissues from injury.

There is experimental evidence that therapeutic levels of ultrasound can induce cavitation in vivo.[23] Acoustic imaging has been used to demonstrate that standard ultrasonic therapy machines can produce detectable gas bubbles in the guinea pig leg, mainly at intermuscular interfaces; these bubbles are presumed to represent ultrasonically induced cavitation events, for they are not produced when irradiation is carried out under raised ambient pressure, a condition which tends to suppress cavitation.[24] The intensity (SATP) threshold for cavitation in vivo is of the order of 0.2 W/cm^2, pulsed 2 msec on: 8 msec off, at 0.75 MHz, and 0.1 W/cm^2 with continuous ultrasound. The position of the nucleation sites at which bubble formation is initiated is not yet known, nor have the conditions necessary for initiation been fully investigated. It must be assumed that the cavitation involved in the studies reported above is of the stable type, for it is difficult to reconcile the therapeutic benefits produced by these levels of treatment with the tissue destruction associated with transient cavitation (see Chapter 3). The gas bubbles involved in transient cavitation undergo irregular oscillations and then implode, producing increases in temperature of thousands of degrees Kelvin and increases in pressure of thousands of atmospheres, localized in regions of only a few microns radius. Any cells exposed to such conditions would clearly be destroyed.

Transient cavitation requires far higher intensities than those used therapeutically[17] and should not occur if ultrasound is administered correctly; the lowest intensity necessary to produce the desired effect should be used, standing-wave conditions should be avoided, and the applicator should be moved continuously throughout treatment. If ultrasound is being used as a heating modality, relatively high intensities will be required (see above); the risk of transient cavitation can be minimized in such conditions by using higher frequencies.[25]

BIOLOGICAL BASIS OF ULTRASONIC THERAPY

Cellular Changes

The intensities and frequencies at which ultrasound is used therapeutically can stimulate cell activity[10] in a manner which could be of fundamental significance to the ultrasonic stimulation of tissue repair.

The cell membrane may well be the primary target for the ultrasonically induced stimulation of cell activity, as it seems to be for other stimulatory agents, for example, pulsating electromagnetic fields.[26] Perturbation of the cell membrane by forces such as those involved in acoustic streaming, possibly in the presence of stable cavitation, could lead to changes in ionic permeability and second messenger activity, which in turn could result in therapeutically advantageous changes such as increased synthesis of protein,[10] increased secretion,[27] and motility changes.[19] The observation of an ultrasonically induced increase in the uptake of calcium ions, known to act as second messengers, after treatment with levels of ultrasound in the therapeutic range,[19] supports this hypothesis.

Tissue Changes

Many of these are a direct result of the local nonthermal changes which ultrasonic irradiation induces in cell activity, although there may also be alteration of connective tissue fiber characteristics after treatment at levels that induce significant increase in temperature.[4]

The relationship of tissue changes to two aspects of ultrasonic therapy, namely, the stimulation of wound healing and of bone repair, will be considered as examples.

Wound Healing

There is now considerable evidence that the healing of a variety of skin injuries, including pressure sores[9, 28] varicose ulcers,[7] and sutured incised wounds[29] can be accelerated and/or mechanically improved by treatment with ultrasound. It has been found that all three of the overlapping phases into which tissue repair is conventionally divided, namely inflammation, proliferation, and remodeling, can be affected by ultrasonic therapy.

During the acute inflammatory phase, mast cells, polymorphonuclear leucocytes, and macrophages migrate to the site of injury where, as a result of wound factor release and phagocytic activity, the repair process is stimulated and the area around the injury site cleared of debris. It has been found that a single treatment with therapeutic ultrasound in vivo can stimulate histamine release from mast cells.[27] If the release of other wound factors from mast cells and macrophages is stimulated, then this may, in part, explain the value of ultrasonic therapy in the early stages of repair. Possibly perturbation of the cell membrane, followed by an increase in second messenger activity, produces this effect. Early release of the wound factors which trigger the subsequent phases of repair should accelerate the onset of those phases. Another change which has been observed when ultrasound is applied shortly after injury is a reduction in local edema.[13] The cause of this reduction has not yet been elucidated.

More is known about the effects of ultrasonic therapy on the second phase of soft tissue repair, proliferation. The main event of this phase is the production of granulation tissue by fibroblasts and endothelial cells which migrate into the wound area from adjacent tissues or proliferate at the injury site. Migration and proliferation are both probably responses to locally released wound factors. Once the granulation tissue begins formation, some of its fibroblasts develop into contractile cells, termed *myofibroblasts,* which initiate wound contraction. The irradiation of fibroblasts with therapeutic ultrasound is followed by changes which are consistent with an increase in the rate of repair,[10, 19, 30] when treatments are given in the proliferative phase. One particularly significant observation is that ultrasonic irradiation at therapeutic levels increases the capacity of fibroblasts to synthesize and secrete the precursors of collagen, the fibrous protein which contributes so much to the development of wound strength.[31] Other changes induced in fibroblasts by therapeutic levels of ultrasound include modification of locomotor activity and temporary increases of intracellular calcium ion levels.[19] All these changes can be suppressed by irradiation at increased pressure, suggesting that cavitation, presumably of the stable type, is involved in their production.[19, 31] The enhanced microstreaming associated with bubble formation could play a part in these changes by affecting the permeability of the cell membrane and promoting the diffusion of ions, dissolved gases, and nutrients.

Ultrasonic treatment during the proliferative phase may stimulate repair in an additional manner, by modifying the microvascular hemodynamics of the wound and adjacent tissue. Improved blood flow has been demonstrated in the arterioles of chronically ischemic muscle after treatment with ultrasound on alternate days for either 1 week or 3 weeks following ligation of the main arterial supply to the muscle. One-megahertz ultrasound, pulsed 100 μsec on:100 μsec off, at an intensity of 2.5 W/cm^2 (SPTA) was applied for 5 minutes at each treatment. The improved blood flow was associated primarily with increased capillary density in the irradiated muscle, compared with that in chronically ischemic but nonirradiated controls, and it was concluded that long-term treatment could improve perfusion in vascularly impaired tissue.[8] If therapeutic levels of ultrasound produce similar effects in granulation tissue, then the increased local perfusion may be yet another factor in the stimulation of repair.

There is some evidence that ultrasonic therapy can affect wound contraction, the reduction of all or part of a skin defect by the centripetal movement of the surrounding skin. Reduction of the size of the wound in this way reduces the need for scar tissue production. Wound contraction begins in the inflammatory phase and extends into the proliferative phase. Myofibroblasts[32] are probably mainly responsible for it, and once achieved the contracted state is maintained by the deposition of collagen fibres. Myofibroblasts are very similar to smooth muscle cells antigenically and ultrastructurally, and since the contraction of smooth muscle cells can be induced by therapeutic levels of ultrasound,[33] it is perhaps not surprising to find that wound contraction, caused primarily by myofibroblast contraction, can be stimulated by similar treatment.[15]

The proliferative phase is succeeded by remodeling, when granulation tissue is gradually replaced by scar tissue, a highly collagenous material with a low cell content and poor blood supply. Over a period of many months, and sometimes years, the pattern in which the replacement collagen fibers is laid down is gradually reshaped by a slow but continuous process into, ideally, one with similar mechanical properties to those of the original uninjured tissue. In practice, where the site of injury is the skin, this is never achieved, the scar tissue remaining weaker and less elastic than the skin indefinitely. It has been found that treatment with therapeutic levels of ultrasound in the first 2 weeks after injury can improve the mechanical properties of skin when examined in the subsequent remodeling stage. The irradiated lesions become slightly stronger and more elastic than do controls, but remain far inferior to uninjured skin.[34]

The collagen fiber pattern of the scar tissue which develops in the irradiated lesions differs from that of controls in that more fiber bundles appear to be present, but each bundle is finer. The presence of more collagen in the scar tissue of treated lesions has been confirmed by biochemical estimation,[31] and the increase in its amount may be related to the slightly higher tensile strength found after a course of treatments with ultrasound. Some of the specimens examined had collagen fibers arranged in a fine lattice pattern after treatment with ultrasound; variation in fiber pattern may be related to the increase in elasticity found but this has yet to be demonstrated. It has been suggested that the development of a collagen lattice in which the fiber angle could change according to the direction in which a tensile force were applied to it could allow a measure of extension and recoil which would increase the amount of energy which could be absorbed by the scar tissue before rupture.[35] It is possible that ultrasonic treatment of mature scar tissue may increase the rate of remodeling of the collagen, so that the initial apparently haphazard arrangement is replaced by one more appropriate to the forces to which the tissue is subjected. This possibility is the subject of current investigation.

To summarize, it would appear that treatment of skin lesions with therapeutic ultrasound at the various stages in their repair can stimulate this repair and improve somewhat the mechanical performance of the resulting scar tissue. The optimum dosage and time of treatment remain to be determined.

Bone Repair

As in soft tissue repair, the repair of bone fractures consists of three overlapping phases of inflammation, proliferation, and remodeling. Furthermore, similar cells, namely mast cells, polymorphonuclear leucocytes, macrophages, fibroblasts, and endothelial cells, are involved in the early stages of both repair processes. Similarities such as these suggest that it should be possible to use therapeutic levels of ultrasound to stimulate bone repair as well as soft tissue repair, and it has recently been shown that this is indeed possible.[11] It has been found that fibular fractures show accelerated repair when treated in the inflammatory and early proliferative phases of repair. Under the conditions of irradiation used [1.5-MHz or 3-MHz ultrasound, pulsed 2 msec on:8 msec off, at an intensity (SATP) of 0.5W/cm² for 5 minutes four times each week] it was found that bone repair tended to be juvenile in type, involving rapid ossification with little cartilage production when irradiation was limited to this period. A more detailed study is now in progress and once this is completed the effect of ultrasound on the repair of weight-bearing bones such as the tibia will be investigated. Preliminary work suggests that ultrasound may have a valuable role to play in the treatment of bone fractures, and could be of considerable value clinically.

CONTRAINDICATIONS AND PRECAUTIONS ASSOCIATED WITH ULTRASONIC THERAPY

Although ultrasonic therapy has an impressive record of safety when correctly used, its very effectiveness as a means of modifying the behavior of cells and tissues makes it a potentially dangerous modality if used inappropriately. A recent publication[36] lists the following as possible contraindications and precautions: the pregnant uterus, the gonads and the structures associated with them, malignancies and precancerous lesions, tissues previously treated by deep x-ray or other radiation, vascular abnormalities including deep vein thrombosis, emboli, and severe atherosclerosis (excluding varicose ulcers), pulmonary tuberculosis and acute infections in general, the cardiac area in advanced heart disease, the eye, the stellate ganglion, hemophiliacs not covered by factor replacement, insonation over bony subcutaneous prominences, epiphyseal plates, the spinal cord after laminectomy, subcutaneous major nerves, the cranium, anesthetic areas, and use of a stationary applicator technique. The size of this list and the sparseness of experimental data suggests that it may be based, at least in part, on the premise that if there is any even unproven fear that damage could ensue, then this should be expressed as a contraindication or a precaution. It is this generally praiseworthy attitude which has helped to give ultrasound such a good safety record,[2] but it may also lead to unnecessary deprivation of some groups of potential patients of effective treatment of injuries and of pain relief. Careful investigations into the rationale of some of the listed contraindications and precautions may well lead to their deletion. An example of such an investigation is that conducted by Magee under the supervision of Reid in 1975.[37] Before this investigation it was often stated that ultrasound had an effect on blood sugar levels and that for this reason the treatment of diabetic patients was contraindicated. In carefully controlled experiments, Magee was unable to find any evidence of a blood sugar alteration after treatment with therapeutic levels of ultrasound, negating the evidence on which this contraindication was based. Although a cautious approach to any form of therapy is always advisable, many of the potentially harmful changes which ultrasound in the therapeutic range might produce can be minimized, and its potentially beneficial effects maximized, if the following procedure is adhered to:

1. Use the lowest intensity consistent with producing the desired therapeutic effect.

2. Move the applicator constantly throughout treatment, to avoid the effects of standing waves.

3. Never treat anesthetic areas.

4. If the patient feels any additional pain during treatment, cease irradiation immediately.

5. Never irradiate the pregnant uterus with therapeutic levels of ultrasound.

6. If in any doubt, do not irradiate.

When properly used, ultrasonic therapy is a most effective means of stimulating a wide range of repair processes, and is thus of considerable clinical value, both actual and potential. The biological basis of its therapeutic effects, and the physical mechanisms by which they are produced, warrant further investigation, for it is only when these are properly understood that it will become possible to use ultrasonic therapy with maximal effectiveness and minimal risk.

ACKNOWLEDGMENTS

I wish to thank my colleagues at Guy's Hospital for their collaboration in many of the experimental investigations referred to in this communication, the physiotherapists who have provided me with so much invaluable information and assistance, and the Medical Research Council, Guy's Arthritis Research Unit, Johnson & Johnson, and the National Fund for Research into Crippling Diseases (grants nos. A/8/1017 and A/8/1153) for financial support of much of the work described.

REFERENCES

1. Dyson M, Suckling J: Stimulation of tissue repair by ultrasound: a survey of the mechanisms involved. Physiotherapy 64:105, 1978
2. Environmental Health Directorate: Canada-wide survey of nonionizing radiation emitting devices. Part II. Ultrasound devices. Report 80–EHD–53. Environmental Health Directorate, Health Protection Branch, Ottawa, Canada, 1980
3. Lele PP, Pierce AD: The thermal hypothesis of the mechanism of ultrasonic focal destruction in organized tissues. p. 121. In Reid JM, Sikov MR (eds): Interaction of Ultrasound and Biological Tissues. Department of Health, Education and Welfare Publication (FDA) 73–8008 BRH/DBE73–1. Rockville, MD, 1972
4. Lehmann JF, Guy AW: Ultrasound therapy. p. 141. In Reid JM, Sikov MR (eds): Interaction of Ultrasound and Biological Tissues. Department of Health, Education and Welfare Publication (FDA) 73–8008 BRH/DBE73–1. Rockville, MD, 1972
5. ter Haar GR, Hopewell JW: Ultrasonic heating of mammalian tissues *in vivo*. Br J Cancer, 45: suppl. V, 65, 1982
6. Dyson M, Joseph J, Pond J, Warwick R: The stimulation of tissue regeneration by means of ultrasound. Clin Sci 35:273, 1968
7. Dyson M, Franks C, Suckling J: Stimulation of healing of varicose ulcers by ultrasound. Ultrasonics 14:232, 1976
8. Hogan RD, Burke KM, Franklin TD: The effect of ultrasound on microvascular hemodynamics in skeletal muscle: effects during ischemia. Microvasc Res 23:370, 1982
9. Paul BJ, La Fratta CW, Dawson AR, et al: Use of ultrasound in the treatment of pressure sores in patients with spinal nerve injury. Arch Phys Med Rehab 41:438, 1960
10. Webster DF, Pond JB, Dyson M, Harvey W: The role of cavitation in the *in vitro* stimulation of protein synthesis in human fibroblasts by ultrasound. Ultrasound Med Biol 4:343, 1978
11. Dyson M, Brookes M: Stimulation of bone repair by ultrasound. p. 61. In Lerski RA, Morley P (eds): Ultrasound '82, Proceedings 3rd Meeting World Federation of Ultrasound in Medicine and Biology. Pergamon Press, Oxford, 1983
12. Griffin JE: Phonophoresis: a review. p. 180. In Mortimer A, Lee N (eds): Proceedings Interna-

tional Symposium on Therapeutic Ultrasound. Canadian Physiotherapy Association, Winnipeg, Canada, 1981

13. Summer W, Patrick MK: Ultrasonic Therapy. A Textbook for Physiotherapists. Elsevier, Amsterdam, London, New York, 1964

14. Dyson M: Non-thermal cellular effects of ultrasound. Br J Cancer, 45: suppl. V, 165, 1982

15. Dyson M: The effect of ultrasound on the rate of wound healing and the quality of scar tissue. p. 110. In Mortimer A, Lee N (eds): Proceedings International Symposium on Therapeutic Ultrasound. Canadian Physiotherapy Association, Winnipeg, Canada, 1981

16. Nyborg WL: Ultrasonic microstreaming and related phenomena. Br J Cancer, 45: suppl. V, 156, 1982

17. Apfel RE: Acoustic cavitation: a possible consequence of biomedical uses of ultrasound. Br J Cancer, 45: suppl. V, 140, 1982

18. Mortimer AJ: Effects of ultrasound on membrane electrophysiology. p. 67. In Mortimer A, Lee N (eds): Proceedings International Symposium on Therapeutic Ultrasound. Canadian Physiotherapy Association, Winnipeg, Canada, 1981

19. Mummery CL: The effect of ultrasound on fibroblasts *in vitro*. Ph.D. thesis, University of London, 1978

20. Farmer WC: Effects of intensity of ultrasound on conduction of motor axons. Phys Ther 48:1233, 1968

21. Madsen PW, Gersten JW: The effects of ultrasound on conduction velocity of peripheral nerve. Arch Phys Med Rehab 42:645, 1961

22. Mortimer AJ, Roy OZ, Trollope BJ, et al: A relationship between ultrasonic intensity and change in myocardial mechanics. Cand J Physiol Pharmacol 58:67, 1980

23. ter Haar G, Daniels S, Eastaugh KC, Hill CR: Ultrasonically induced cavitation *in vivo*. Br J Cancer, 45: suppl. V, 151, 1982

24. Morton KI: The role of non-thermal mechanisms in the interaction of ultrasound with biological systems. Ph.D. thesis, University of London, 1982

25. Flynn HG: Generation of transient cavities in liquids by microsecond pulses of ultrasound. J Acoust Soc Am 72:1926, 1982

26. Johnson DE, Rodan GA: The effect of pulsating electromagnetic fields on prostaglandin synthesis in osteoblast-like cells. Trans 2nd Annual Meeting Bioelectrical Repair and Growth Society, 2:7, Oxford, England, Sept. 20–22, 1982

27. Fyfe MC, Chahl, LA: Mast cell degranulation. A possible mechanism of action of therapeutic ultrasound. Ultrasound Med Biol, 8: suppl. I, 62, 1982 (abstr)

28. McDiarmid T: A study by means of a double-blind randomised controlled trial to determine the effect of therapeutic ultrasound on the healing time of superficial pressure sores. M.Sc. thesis, University of Southampton, England, 1982

29. Drastichova V, Samohyl J, Slavetinska W: Strengthening of sutured skin wounds with ultrasound in experiments in animals. Acta Chir Plast (Praha) 15:114, 1973

30. Harvey W, Dyson M, Pond JB, Grahame R: The *in vivo* stimulation of protein synthesis in human fibroblasts by therapeutic levels of ultrasound. Proceedings 2nd European Congress on Ultrasonics in Medicine. Amsterdam, Excerpta Medica Int Cong Ser 363:10, 1975

31. Webster DF: The effect of ultrasound on wound healing. Ph.D. thesis, University of London, 1980

32. Gabbiani G, Hirschel BJ, Ryan GB, et al: Granulation tissue as a contractile organ. J Exp Med 135:719, 1972

33. ter Haar G, Dyson M, Talbert D: Ultrasonically induced contraction in mouse uterine smooth muscle *in vivo*. Ultrasonics 16:275, 1978

34. Dyson M: Stimulation of tissue repair by therapeutic ultrasound. p. 206. In Dineen P, Hildick-Smith G (eds): The Surgical Wound. Lea and Febiger, Philadelphia, 1981

35. Forrester JC: Mechanical, biochemical and architectural features of surgical repair. Adv Biol Med Phys 14:1, 1973

36. Reid DC: Possible contraindications and precautions associated with ultrasound therapy. p. 274. In Mortimer A, Lee N (eds): Proceedings International Symposium on Therapeutic Ultrasound. Canadian Physiotherapy Association, Winnipeg, 1981

37. Magee DJ: The effect of therapeutic ultrasound on the level of blood sugar in the human body. M.Sc. thesis, University of Alberta, Canada, 1975

12 Local Hyperthermia by Ultrasound for Cancer Therapy

PADMAKAR P. LELE

From the data collected by the National Cancer Institute's Surveillance, Epidemiology and End Result Program it is estimated that there will be 1,320,000 new cancer patients in the United States in 1984. During the same period, 450,000 patients will die from cancer despite surgery, radiation therapy, chemotherapy, and immunotherapy. These numbers underline the need for development and deployment of additional effective anticancer modalities. Hyperthermia, at temperatures above 41°C has been used sporadically in treatment of cancer apparently since 2,000 B.C. In this century the results, though often dramatically successful were generally inconsistent, presumably through a lack of adequate technology for production of predictable and controllable hyperthermia. The current resurgence of interest stems from the emphatic demonstration of significant tumoricidal effects of hyperthermia in patients in whom all conventional modes of therapy had failed. Concurrently, laboratory studies have provided the scientific rationale for its use based on demonstrably greater heat sensitivity of malignant tumors than normal tissues, and, to a lesser extent, of malignant or transformed cells as compared with normal cells. In this chapter we will briefly summarize the biological basis for the tumoricidal action of hyperthermia and then discuss the use of ultrasound for local tumor hyperthermia. Further information on the various aspects of hyperthermia can be found in the several publications now available.[1-6]

Although there is a difference in the heat sensitivities of malignant and normal tissues (and cells) it is rather small. Furthermore, studies on cell cultures in vitro indicate that a small difference in heat dose (temperature-duration history) produces a large difference in the numbers of cells killed. Thus, to minimize the toxicity to normal tissues and to maximize it to the tumor mass, heating must be localized to the predetermined target volume, as well as be precisely controllable.

At high temperatures and/or long durations, hyperthemia can cause coagulation pan-necrosis of tissues. At lower heat-dose levels, hyperthermia leads to reproductive arrest of the multiplying cells as well as to changes in local blood perfusion. Hyperthermia affects cells in the S phase of the cell cycle, has preferentially greater effect on hypoxic, acidic (low pH), and malnourished cells, all of which tend to be radioresistant. Thus, hyperthermia can be synergistic with radiation therapy, or at least produce an additive effect. It can also enhance the cytotoxicity of chemotherapeutic agents both directly from the higher temperature and also, under appropriate conditions, indirectly through increased blood perfusion.

Preliminary clinical data appear to confirm and justify the results obtained in cell cultures and animal studies. Temperatures of 42.5°C or higher for 20–30 minutes appear to be necessary for tumoricidal effects, and several sessions—preferably at intervals of 2 or more days—seem to be required for significant tumor regression. High incidence of serious toxicity related to damage and/or dysfunction of the central nervous system, liver, kidney, and heart precludes routine use of temperatures above about 41.5°C for whole body (or systemic) hyperthermia. Regional perfusion hyperthermia of extremities when combined with an appropriate drug such as melphalan has yielded striking results in disseminated lesions such as melanomas. There is, however, a risk of damage to the perfused artery from the hot perfusate, and the technique cannot be applied to the trunk and the head and neck regions. These restrictions do not apply to localized hyperthermia. In principle, any effective tumoricidal heat-dose could be delivered to the target volume without any damage or toxicity to nontarget tissues if the heating can be truly localized to the target tissue regardless of its depth or location. Such localized hyperthermia alone or in combination with radiation therapy or drugs could be an effective anticancer modality, since local failure is believed to be the cause of death in 65–75 percent of cancer patients.

In production of local hyperthermia for cancer therapy, noninvasiveness of the technique is of great importance since disruption of lymphatics and blood vessels and mechanical probing of the tumor might increase metastasization. Ultrasonic and electromagnetic (EM) radiations are the two principal modalities potentially useful for this purpose.

PLANE WAVE FIELDS

The volume, extent, and uniformity of the hyperthermia are governed by the pattern of heat generation in the tissues and of heat diffusion from conduction and blood flow. Since heat diffusion in circumscribed tissue volumes cannot effectively be controlled, the optimization of the technique for production of uniform, controllable hyperthermia relies almost entirely on the control over the pattern of heat generation in the tissues by the modality used.

Let us consider the pattern of heat generation in tissues by EM fields and ultrasound. If a uniform intensity field of any form of radiant energy were to impinge upon a medium with uniform attenuation and thermal characteristics

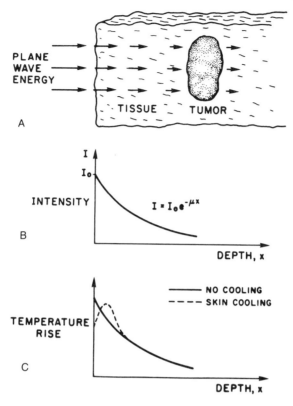

FIG. 12.1 Intensity and temperature distribution patterns in a homogeneous medium with plane wave radiation (see text).

(Fig. 12.1A), the intensity would decay exponentially with increasing depth in the medium (Fig. 12.1B). And since, for a given absorption coefficient, the rate of heat generation is proportional to the local intensity, it would also decay exponentially with depth. Given uniform thermal properties—specific heat, heat conduction, and heat transport by blood flow—the pattern of temperature distribution would also be similar, being highest at the surface and decaying exponentially with depth (Fig. 12.1C). In the case of biological tissues in vivo, it is not possible to compensate for this gradient of temperature, to any useful extent, by cooling of the skin. Cooling, on the other hand, may cause elevation of subcutaneous temperatures from the resulting vasoconstriction (Fig. 12.1C). Attenuation of ultrasonic or EM energy in transit through an attenuating medium is directly related to the frequency employed. Therefore, for a given intensity at the surface, less energy is lost in transit to a given depth in the medium, and higher local intensities are obtained at lower frequencies than at higher frequencies. But note that energy not attenuated in the target volume and overlying tissues will be transmitted into deeper tissues and may undergo multiple reflections, refraction and scattering until it is absorbed completely, since it cannot leave the body. Thus, for instance, if a frequency of 0.3 MHz is used to heat a tumor 10 cm below the surface, almost 80 percent of the incident energy will be transmitted deeper and lead to the heating of deeper tissue, especially of soft tissue-bone interfaces.

The same considerations apply to situations in which the source, a radiofrequency (RF) or microwave antenna or ultrasound transducer, is placed intraluminally within a cavity or interstitially in the tumor. The intensity and temperature rise will be highest at the probe-tissue interface and decay exponentially at increasing distances. Studies conducted in the author's laboratory indicate that for therapeutically effective heating such probes may need to be placed 10–12 mm apart, making this technique clinically unacceptable for production of hyperthermia per se. However, if radioactive sources are implanted for interstitial radiotherapy, they could as well be utilized for delivery of local hyperthermia for enhancing the therapeutic effect.

MULTIPLE BEAM SUPERPOSITION

One of the ways in which higher intensities could be obtained at depth compared to those at the surface, is by superposition at the target volume of two or more beams entering the medium through different portals. Rotation of the source of energy in an arc centered at the deep target is commonly practiced in radiation therapy to deliver a higher total dose to a deep target than to the intervening tissues. Superposition of multiple beams of electromagnetic or ultrasonic energy, however, poses serious problems of phasing. In the regions where they are out of phase, they would interfere destructively and the local intensity (and the consequent heat generation) may be significantly lower than in the individual beams. It is also well to bear in mind that the intensity in each beam will decay exponentially from the surface inwards. The maximum depth at which a "dose" higher than that at the surface could be achieved would be dependent upon both the attenuation characteristics of the intervening tissues and the portal/target area ratio. Furthermore, with multiple stationary overlapping beams maximal heating occurs at the points of their intersection as seen in Figure 12.2.

FOCUSED FIELDS

With the use of a focused beam higher intensities and therefore higher temperatures can be achieved at the target at depth as compared with intervening tissues (Fig. 12.3). Specifically, the temperature rise at the surface over the skin, the mucosa or granulation tissue, and the relatively less vascular subcutaneous tissues, can be held to a negligible value. The intensity decays rapidly in tissues beyond the focus, by beam divergence as well as by attenuation, thus minimizing the temperature elevation in tissues, such as bone underlying the tumor.

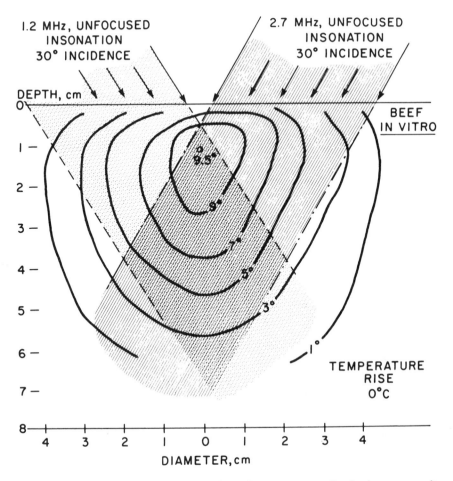

FIG. 12.2 Temperature distribution resulting from two cross-fired, plane wave ultrasound beams, superimposed at the target volume.

CHOICE OF FREQUENCY

Most of the ultrasonic energy that is attenuated in soft tissues is absorbed locally and generates heat. The energy attenuated in tissues superficial to the tumor is thus not only wasteful, but since it generates heat it is also detrimental to the goal of sharply localized heating of the tumor. Attenuation can be reduced by use of a lower frequency but this would also reduce the heat generation within the tumor, requiring proportionately higher intensities to achieve therapeutic temperature levels. The choice of the proper frequency and aperture, crucial for localization of hyperthermia, is thus an exercise in optimization of these conflicting requirements for the size, depth, and the absorption/attenuation properties of each specific tumor and the overlying tissues. These compu-

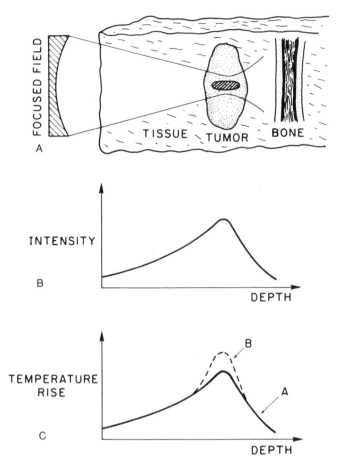

FIG. 12.3 Intensity and temperature distribution patterns with a focused insonation field. C. The solid line represents the pattern of temperature distribution, if the ultrasonic and thermophysical properties of the tumor were the same as those of the tissues. The dashed line represents the pattern of temperature distribution, if the ultrasonic absorption coefficient in the tumor was higher than that of tissues and/or the heat transport in the tumor was lower than that in tissues.

tations are essential ingredients of therapy planning for both ultrasonic and electromagnetic hyperthermia.

The frequency also determines the wavelength and thus the size and shape of the focus and therefore the minimum size of the target volume that can be selectively heated. The focal regions of ultrasonic and EM fields are elongated and are typically five to six wavelengths long. Therefore, the wavelength should not be longer than about 1/6 the "thickness" of the tumor. For heating a spherical tumor 3 cm in diameter, for example, the wavelength probably should not be more than about 5 mm and for a 6-cm-diameter tumor, not more than about 1 cm. For EM waves of these wavelengths, the half-power penetration depths in tissues are only a few millimeters. Localized heating of tumors, situated at depths greater than approximately 14 mm from the skin or the mucous membranes, is thus not possible by EM radiation. Ultrasound, at these wavelengths, can penetrate to the deepest tumors. The wavelength of thermogenic, nonionizing electromagnetic energy that can penetrate to the midplane of the body is so long (15–20 cm) that it produces regional rather than localized heating.

BEAM STEERING AND INTENSITY MODULATION

Focusing concentrates the energy from the transducer into a focal region which serves as a noninvasive heat source within the tissue. The diameter (half-power beam width) of such a focal region may typically be 0.3–3 mm, whereas that of a typical tumor may be 5–10 cm. The focus thus needs to be moved about within different regions of the tumor. The rate of deposition of energy at any region must be adjusted to the local heat removal capacity. It also needs to be higher during induction of hyperthermia than for its sustenance. Considering the time constants of temperature decay in tissues in vivo, the energy deposition at any region must be repeated every 3–10 seconds. The focus thus can be moved about in different regions of the target volume over this period. It is also necessary to modulate the intensity at the transducer to compensate for differences in path lengths and attenuation in the tissues overlying different regions of the target volume.

It is not necessary to distribute the energy evenly throughout the entire target volume for induction of uniform temperature elevation. As a matter of fact, such uniform energy deposition would lead to nonhomogeneous temperature distribution as shown in Figure 12.4A. The periphery of the target volume, through which heat is lost to the surrounding "normothermic" tissues by conduction and blood flow, would necessarily be cooler than the central region. But, since the tumor grows at its margin and infiltrates the tumor bed tissues, it is at this location that the temperature must be therapeutically adequate. Therefore, more energy needs to be delivered at the periphery than in the inner regions (Fig. 12.4B). It is indeed possible to induce uniform hyperthermia in target volumes up to approximately 20 mm in diameter by deposition of heat at the periphery alone. In larger volumes, a small proportion of energy needs to be deposited in the central region to heat it to a therapeutic temperature. Such control over the pattern and magnitude of energy deposition in tumors which are irregular in shape requires the use of a computer. A computer-controlled, steered, intensity-modulated, focused ultrasound system was developed and evaluated extensively in animal tissues in vitro and in vivo, in transplanted murine tumors, and in spontaneous tumors in dog and human patients in the author's laboratory. In addition to its capability to deliver uniform dose distributions in tissues and tumors in which it has been evaluated, it is also unique in its capability to selectively heat desired target volumes located at depth, noninvasively, and without unacceptable or significant temperature elevation in tissues overlying or surrounding the target volume. Details on the

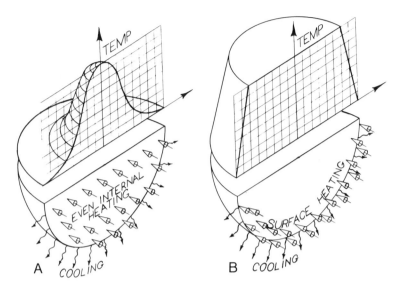

FIG. 12.4 Temperature distributions in a tissue volume resulting from deposition of energy (A) uniformly through its volume and (B) preferentially on its surface.

design and operation of the system can be found in previous publications.[7-12] Based on the clinical experience with this system, an electronically steered phased array is presently under development and evaluation.

ENERGY REQUIREMENTS

An approximate estimate of the energy requirements for heating a given target may be obtained by assuming it to have the same thermophysical properties as water and a volume larger than the target by a factor proportional to the average (or estimated) blood flow for the target tissue. Typically, blood flow may impose an additional heat load equivalent to 70 percent of the target volume. The ultrasonic power needed to raise the temperature of a tumor with "typical" blood flow, 6 cm in diameter and with an intensity absorption coefficient of 0.3 dB/cm/MHz[12-14] by 7°C in 10 minutes using 1-MHz ultrasound, can be calculated to be approximately 10 watts. If the tumor was situated at a depth of 6 cm, and the overlying tissue had the same ultrasonic absorption (attenuation) characteristics as the tumor, approximately 15 watts of power will be needed at the portal. If a 1-MHz, 6-cm-diameter transducer focused at 12 cm was used for heating this tumor, the spatial average intensity would be approximately 20 W/cm² with a spatial peak intensity of approximately 60 W/cm².

AVOIDANCE OF COLLAPSE CAVITATION

Such acoustic power requirements for induction of hyperthermia might lead to cavitation damage because of the high peak intensities if sharp focusing were used. Special "smeared focus" lenses, in which peak intensities are lowered without compromising the angle of beam convergence, were therefore designed. The peak intensities employed for production of hyperthermia are always well below the threshold for cavitation-induced damage in organized mammalian tissues.[15] Extensive theoretical and experimental research on ultrasonically induced cavitation and damage thresholds in mammalian tissues in vitro and in vivo conducted in this laboratory shows that although stable bubble-oscillation type of cavitation occurs even at intensity levels associated with diagnostic ultrasound, transient collapse-cavitation resulting in structural damage does not occur in organized tissues until peak focal intensity is higher than 1,450 W/cm² at 2- to 3-MHz frequency. Occurrence of transient cavitation was invariably associated with occurrence of tissue damage but no damage was ever found to occur with bubble-oscillation type of cavitation unless it was induced by temperature elevation. Thresholds for both types of cavitation are known to be lower at lower frequencies in liquid media, and in the absence of definitive information are presumed to be similarly lower in organized tissues.

TEMPERATURE DISTRIBUTIONS PRODUCED BY STATIONARY OR STEERED BEAMS OF UNFOCUSED OR FOCUSED ULTRASOUND IN PHANTOMS AND TISSUES IN VITRO AND IN VIVO

Temperature distributions resulting from insonation with stationary and steered beams of unfocused or focused ultrasound were measured in tissue-equivalent phantoms, beef muscle in vitro, and in dog muscle mass, and several types of transplanted murine tumors in vivo. In some experiments in vivo, a live, anesthetized rat bearing a $10 \times 10 \times 10$-cm tumor was placed inside the abdomen of an anesthetized dog to simulate a deep-seated, large tumor. Arrays of four to six thermocouples 25–125 μm in diameter, stepped under computer control in submillimeter steps through the volume of interest, were used to measure the steady-state temperatures at 600–800 locations in both in vitro and in vivo experiments. Confirmation of results was sought in spontaneous tumors in dog patients in vivo, using fewer multijunction thermocouple probes. Detailed results are published elsewhere.[9-12] Salient features are summarized below.

PLANE WAVE ULTRASOUND

In normal tissues (Fig. 12.5) as well as in tumors, insonation with plane wave ultrasound, 0.6–6.0 MHz in frequency, results in spatially nonuniform hyperthermia which is characterized by the existence of a small, almost punctate, region of maximum temperature rise, the depth of which appears to be dependent on the absorption coefficient and heat transfer properties of the medium and cannot be altered by spatial manipulation of the plane wave ultrasonic source. The existence of an ultrasound-reflecting structure below the target may lead to the generation of a second region of hyperthermia at depth. The region of maximum temperature elevation is eccentric relative to the transducer and, due to the smallness of its size, it cannot be easily located except by thorough scanning of the region in all three orthogonal planes. It is thus likely to be missed by temperature measuring procedures practicable under clinical conditons. This may explain the occurrence of burns observed by various investigators in animal and human tumor treatments using plane wave ultrasound.[16, 17] Furthermore, the resultant nonuniformity of temperature distributions within the target volume (Fig. 12.5B) renders impossible any precise correlation of the temperature and duration of hyperthermia (either alone or in combination with radiation or chemotherapy) with resultant effects on tumors. Plane wave ultrasound is thus not optimal even for therapy of superficial lesions.

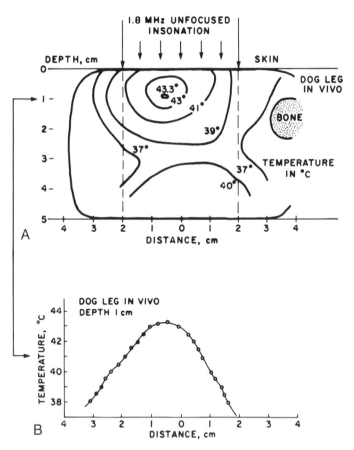

FIG. 12.5 Steady-state temperature distribution in the gluteal muscle mass of dog in vivo from plane wave 1.8-MHz ultrasound. A. Isotherms plotted from temperatures measured at 1-mm spacing along nine tracks. B. The temperature distribution along the track at 1-cm depth.

STEERED, FOCUSED ULTRASOUND

All the above problems and difficulties are obviated by use of steered, focused, and intensity-modulated ultrasound which enables precise tailoring of the heat dose to individual tumors. Spatially uniform levels of hyperthermia, restricted to the target volume (Fig. 12.6), located superficially or at depth can be achieved. Details on the controllable and selective deep heating by this technique in comparison with cross-fired and isocentric systems have been published elsewhere.[10-12]

The ability to heat a discrete tumor volume at depth to a uniform hyperthermia temperature has the advantages of (1) sparing of overlying and adjacent normal tissues, and (2) uniform treatment field dosage. The latter is essential for establishing temperature/duration relationships with any accuracy, whether for tumor response or underlying biological mechanisms, for hyperthermia alone, or with radiation or chemotherapy.

PRELIMINARY STUDIES ON TUMOR TEMPERATURE DISTRIBUTION IN TRANSPLANTED MURINE TUMORS

Tumor-bearing rodents were used in large numbers for comparison of different ultrasonic methods for production of hyperthermia and for optimization of the steered, intensity modulated, focused ultrasound system. Although tumor regression was observed in almost all of the animals, in those exposed to plane wave ultrasound it was not possible to correlate the magnitude of tumor regression with the temperature and duration (heat-dose), since the stepped thermocouple technique revealed that different parts of the tumor were subjected to different levels of hyperthermia. It was also observed that many of the tumors thus treated appeared to develop the shape of a crater (occasionally with central ulceration as previously reported by Marmor et al.[16, 17] suggesting that tumor regression in the central area was accompanied by continued tumor growth at the periphery. By contrast, with steered, focused ultrasound tumor regression was found to occur with two or three weekly sessions at 43°C and appeared to be uniform across the entire treated area. Data from all these animals, used primarily for studies on distribution of hyperthermia, have not been used for deducing quantitative dose-effect relationships because of the large numbers of thermocouple-probes which had repeatedly been inserted and retracted through the tumor. Results of a dose-effect study[18] conducted after standardization of the technique and use of one or two multijunction thermocouple probes are shown in Figure 12.7.

SPONTANEOUS TUMORS IN DOG PATIENTS

Thirteen dogs with inoperable or recurrent, biopsy-proven malignant tumors were treated with ultrasonic hyperthermia, alone or with radiation. Local hy-

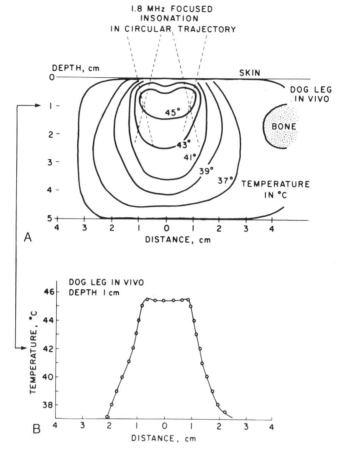

FIG. 12.6 Steady-state temperature distribution in the gluteal muscle mass of dog in vivo from steered, intensity-modulated focused 1.8-MHz ultrasound. A. Isotherms plotted from temperatures measured at 1-mm spacing along nine tracks. B. The temperature distribution along the track at 1-cm depth. Note the uniformity of temperature distribution within and the sharp fall-off of temperature outside the hyperthermia field. By contrast to hyperthermia by plane wave ultrasound in the same preparation, shown in Figure 12.5, note the absence of any reflective heating at the depth of 3.5 cm.

perthermia at a temperature 42.5–43°C for 20 minutes was given once a week for 3–6 weeks and in some instances was combined with 600–660 rad of superficial x-radiation (100 kVp, 8mA). In large, rapidly growing, mucosal or submucosal tumors with a natural drainage portal in the oral cavity or the aerodigestive tract, causing difficulty in eating, swallowing, or respiration, in vivo cytoreduction of 25–33 percent of tumor volume was accomplished by focal coagulation. The combinations of temperature and duration were selected with reference to the extensive data on local heat tolerance of normal mammalian tissues including man in vivo,[19] shown in Figure 12.8. Different temperature-duration

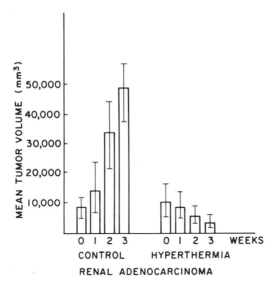

FIG. 12.7   Effect of local hyperthermia at 43°C for 20 minutes, once a week, on the growth of renal adenocarcinoma in the rat. Studies were started 4 weeks after implantation of tumor.

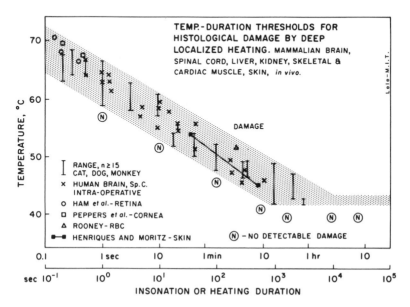

FIG. 12.8   Temperature-duration thresholds for histologic damage by localized heating at depth of mammalian tissues in vivo.

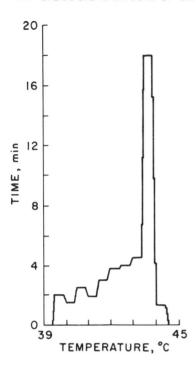

FIG. 12.9   Time-temperature histogram of a hyperthermia therapy session in a dog patient.

combinations were selected along the lower edge of the plotted data to test their equivalence in causing coagulation necrosis of the tumor tissue leading to nonhemorrhagic cytoreduction. The procedure was repeated in other regions of the tumor with an interval of 1–2 weeks, and was followed by tumor-bed hyperthermia. The dogs were anesthetized with nitrous oxide-halothane anesthesia delivered intratracheally for the treatments. One or two multi-thermocouple probes placed into the tumor, and two unsheathed probes placed on the surface, were used to monitor temperatures during hyperthermia. One of the thermocouples was placed in contact with the underlying bone, when present. In oral tumors hyperthermia was induced by using an exponential-horn waveguide insonator.[10, 11] Before the end of the prescribed duration of hyperthermia one of the intratumoral thermocouple probes was pulled out in steps of 1 mm to ascertain the intratumoral temperature distribution. The temperature history of the tumor from the beginning to the end of each therapy session was plotted out from the data in the computer to determine the total duration for which the tumor was subjected to each temperature during induction and maintenance of hyperthermia, and cooling to normothermic levels. An example of such a plot is given in Figure 12.9.

RESULTS

Analysis of the strip-chart records of the temperature rise and the insonation power showed that in most, if not all, instances following 3–5 minutes of intratumoral temperature of 43°C there was a sudden drop in temperature, and more insonation power was needed for restitution of the temperature to 43°C. Three to 5 minutes after restitution of this temperature, the power requirements were lower. This phenomenon was similar to that observed in human patients (shown in Fig. 12.13) and possibly denotes a thermovascular response.

The temperature distribution across the tumor plotted from data obtained by pulling out the thermocouple probe in steps of 1 mm or 2 mm, before termination of hyperthermia, showed uniform temperature distribution, with steep fall-off beyond the hyperthermia field in almost all instances, similar to that seen in human patients (Fig. 12.12). The presence of bone underlying the tumor did not seem to perturb the temperature distribution in the tumor. The temperatures measured at the bone surface were the same as those in overlying soft tissues when the tumor was on or within 5 mm of the bone. With tumors separated from the bone by 1 cm or more, the surface temperature at the bone was lower than the intratumoral temperature. Computer-generated histograms of cumulated duration at various temperatures (Fig. 12.9) show that little time was spent at subtherapeutic temperatures during the induction of hyperthermia and during cooling after termination of insonation.

The temperature-duration combination for coagulation necrosis of tumor tissue did not differ greatly from that of normal tissues (Fig. 12.8), although in most instances it was approximately 1°C lower at any given duration.

A change in the color of the tumor was always evident immediately at the end of each treatment which resulted in coagulation necrosis. This was followed by sloughing-off of the tumor coagulum in 6–8 days. With hyperthermia at 42.5°C there was little discernible color change, if any. The entire series of treatments, involving more than 113 insonation sessions, was remarkable for the absence of any unintended toxicity, except in two instances of skin injury resulting from the difficulties in positioning the insonation head using the mechanical focus-indicating pointer system which has since then been replaced by a fiberoptic system. No changes attributable to the treatment were seen in radiographs of the bone in any animals, except in an osteosarcoma.

The oncologic results in this series of patients, small as it was, were as follows:

Four fibrosarcomas and one odontoma showed total regression with hyperthermia alone, but recurred in 6 weeks. After hyperthermia combined with radiation therapy, the patients were disease free for periods ranging from 9 to 18 months. Biopsies showed no tumor cells in the treatment field. Melanomas, melanosarcoma, undifferentiated sarcoma, osteosarcoma, and tonsillar carcinoma responded to hyperthemia alone with enduring local control. All these tumors, except osteosarcoma, were sensitive to hyperthermia at 42.5°C for 30 minutes. There were no metastases to lungs in patients with normal chest radiographs at the initiation of therapy. This fact is specially noteworthy in the case of osteosarcoma, which in dogs metastasizes early to lungs (approximately 12 weeks). With successful treatment of the primary, the dog remained free of lung metastases for 9½ months at which time it was killed for nonmedical reasons. Three of the patients were disease-free 14–30 months after therapy. Others died from nononcologic disease or remote spread of malignancy. No disease was found at autopsy at the site of the primary lesion.

SPONTANEOUS TUMORS IN HUMAN PATIENTS

Feasibility and toxicity studies of local tumor hyperthermia by focused ultrasound in human patients were conducted collaboratively with Dr. Kaiser of Pondville Hospital, Walpole, MA, Dr. Feldman of Boston University Medical Center, Boston, Drs. Frei and Ervin of the Sidney Farber Cancer Institute, Boston, Drs. Bertino and Kowal of Yale–New Haven Hospital, New Haven, CT, and Drs. Shimm and Suit of Massachusetts General Hospital, Boston, under protocols approved by the Human Subjects Committees of the collaborating institutions, the Massachusetts Institute of Technology (MIT), and the MIT Clinical Research Center. A brief summary is presented below. For details please see reference 20.

Initial studies were conducted using two special systems of simplified insonation equipment developed for production of uniform distribution of hyperthermia in small superficial tumors up to 3 cm in diameter. One was a motor-driven system which rotated an insonation head in a circular trajectory of adjustable diameter. The other, a stationary insonator, consisted of an annular focusing system which projected a pattern of intensity distribution similar to that of a focused transducer rotating in a circular trajectory. The transducer could be operated either in continuous-wave or pulsed modes. To increase the diameter of region of uniformity from approximately 20 to about 30 mm a controllable "center leak" was added to the "annular focus" design of the lens.[9] A diagrammatic cross-section through the lens and the intensity distribution are shown in Figure 12.10. The computer-controlled, steered, focused ultrasonic system was used for larger and deeper extracavitary tumors.

The studies were conducted on patients with histologically verified malignant tumors which were refractory to other anticancer modalities. Intratumoral and surface temperatures were measured by 75 μm-diameter thermocouples placed at different depths in the tumor through a 22-gauge hypodermic needle or attached to the skin as shown in Figure 12.11. The depth of the thermocouple was checked by A-mode echography at 15 MHz. Ultrasound hyperthermia was administered to raise the intratumoral temperature to 42.5°C for 20 minutes once each week for 3 weeks. If there was no toxicity and no response after three sessions, the temperature was raised to 43°C for the subsequent three sessions.

Tumor size was measured initially and in follow-up examinations using conventional techniques, CT scans, or ultrasonograms. Skin was examined for erythema, bullae, or breakdown before and after each session. A tumor biopsy was obtained between 12 and 24 weeks posttherapy. If the patient complained of a burning sensation or pain during therapy, the skin was cooled by cooling the water in the coupling bath.

Most of the tumors (30 of 44) treated were over bones, lungs, or the aerodiges-

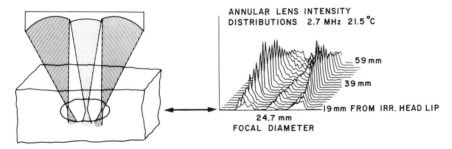

FIG. 12.10 Annular-focus lens with a central "leak": diagrammatic cross-section and intensity distribution.

tive tract, that is, at sites considered to be difficult to heat satisfactorily with ultrasound. A special attempt was made to record the temeprature at the bone or air interfaces whenever feasible. Before the end of the treatment session the intratumoral and surface thermocouple probes were pulled out manually in small steps to determine spatial temperature distribution. Tumor temperature could be raised to the level desired in all tumors studied, except perhaps one. This was a pulsatile, frontal bone osteosarcoma in which measurement of temperature at depth was not advisable because of imprecise information on the location of the meninges and of the tumor vasculature. Intratumoral temperature distributions with the annular focus lens were uniform to ±0.25°C across the hyperthermia volume (Fig. 12.12). With the use of steered, intensity-modulated focused beam, the variation was ±0.1°C. Due to optimization of ultrasonic frequency, focusing characteristics and beam angulation, presence of the bone was found not to distort the intratumoral temperature distribution appreciably, nor was the temperature at the periosteum found to differ by more than ±0.3°C from the intratumoral temperature. None of the patients reported occurrence

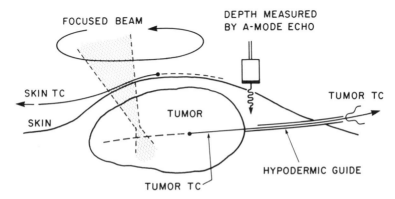

FIG. 12.11 Thermometry procedure in human patients—see text. Annular focus lens was substituted for steered focused beam in part of the study. Coupling water bath is not shown.

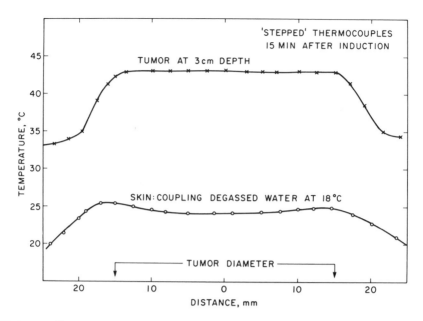

FIG. 12.12 Cutaneous and intratumoral temperature distributions with the use of the annular focus lens.

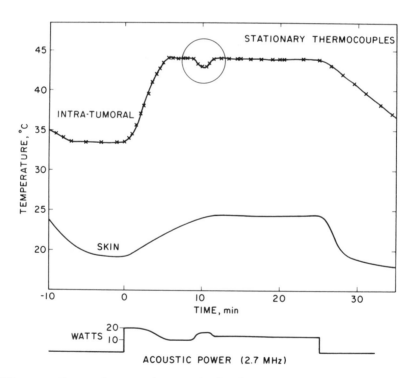

FIG. 12.13 Temporal course of intratumoral and cutaneous temperatures and the acoustical power. The thermovascular response is circled.

of deep-seated pain during hyperthermia. No symptoms or signs of bone damage were reported subsequently, nor was any evidence of bone damage seen in three patients examined radiographically 10–12 weeks after hyperthermia. Intratumoral temperature of 43°C or higher sustained for 3–5 minutes evoked a vasomotor response leading to a drop in the temperature. Increased power was needed to restore the temperature to the previous level (Fig. 12.13). The power required to sustain this temperature became slightly reduced in 3–5 minutes after restoration of the temperature.

Of the 44 patients entered into this study, 7 had diffuse tumors with undefined boundaries. Hyperthermia resulted in subjective and objective improvements in the status of the tumors in five of these seven patients. These included partial relief of pain when previously present, decrease in amount of drugs required for control of pain, reduced trismus, and "flattening" and "shrinkage" of the tumor. But these could not be quantified with confidence. Adequate temperature measurements could not be made in one case (osteosarcoma). These eight patients are excluded from assessment of response to hyperthermia. The results in the 36 remaining patients are shown in Table 12.1.

The highest temperature used was 43°C, except in one patient with a schwannoma in whom it was 45°C at one session. There was no subjective or objective toxicity except as noted in Table 12.1. Some of the patients tended to fall

TABLE 12.1   Reduction in tumor size[a] following ultrasound hyperthermia

		Regression			
Total		0%	<50%	>50%	100%
1	Inflammatory carcinoma of the breast	1			
1	Schwannoma	1[b]			
1	Renal cell carcinoma	1			
2	Acinar cell carcinoma			2	
2	Melanoma				2[c]
3	Undifferentiated sarcoma			1	2
3	Chest wall metastases of breast carcinoma			3	
23	Squamous cell carcinoma	1	6[d]	14	2
36		4	6	20	6

[a] $D_1 \times D_2 \times D_3/2$, where D_1, D_2 and D_3 are 3 perpendicular cross-diameters.
[b] Tumor located in amputation stump and invading skin. Patient reported feeling of "tenseness" within the region lasting approximately 30 hours following hyperthermia. Increase in preexisting "redness" of skin following 45°C for 20 minutes. No change in tumor measurements.
[c] Both tumors disappeared after two sessions at 42.5°C for 20 minutes. Control tumors continued to grow even with concurrent chemotherapy. In one patient there was hemorrhage from multiple sites in control tumors 3 weeks following last hyperthermia.
[d] In one patient with previous neck dissection there was referred pain along the scar which was remote from treatment area. The pain was not dose-limiting.

asleep during hyperthermia and had to be kept awake to prevent any sudden motions on awakening from sleep. The absence of toxicity with the use of this technique is in marked contrast to the pain, blistering, and burning of the skin or "shelling out" of the tumor reported by investigators using plane wave ultrasound[16, 17] and must be attributed to the sparing of tissues outside the target volume by focusing the ultrasonic energy into the tumor.

Maximum response in each patient occurred early in the course of treatments. Partial response (50 percent regression) was obtained in 72 percent (26 of 36) tumors with complete regression in 17 percent (6 of 36) tumors. These results must be viewed in the context that due to the fixed diameter of the field of the annular focus system, only a part was exposed to hyperthermia in patients treated with that system. In eight of the tumors in which the tumor regression was less than 50 percent, biopsy 12–24 weeks after the end of hyperthermia treatments showed absence of viable tumor cells. Thus, even though there was no shrinkage in tumor volume, the malignancy was controlled in these cases. In one tumor, which did not respond, biopsy showed presence of viable tumor cells.

Seven of the patients with multiple tumors were on chemotherapy (two on cis-platinum-bleomycin, two on cyclophosphamide, two on methotrexate, and one on cis-platinum). In these only one tumor was treated with hyperthermia. In five patients the control tumors showed no response to chemotherapy alone, but the tumors treated additionally with hyperthermia showed partial regression. In two patients, the control tumors showed partial regression, while the tumors treated additionally with hyperthermia showed complete regression.

Local hyperthermia by focused, steered, intensity-modulated ultrasound has thus a great potential in cancer therapy, whether used alone or in combination with radiation therapy or/and chemotherapy.

ACKNOWLEDGMENTS

Parts of this research were supported by United States Public Health Service Grants RR00088, CA30944, and CA31303 and Contract No. 1-CM27525.

REFERENCES

1. Streffer C, van Beuningen D, Dietzel F, et al (eds): Cancer Therapy by Hyperthermia and Radiation (Proceedings 2nd International Symposium, Essen, West Germany, June 2–4, 1977). Urban and Schwarzenberg, Baltimore-Munich, 1978

2. Milder JW (ed:) Conference on hyperthermia in cancer treatment. Cancer Res 39:2231, 1979

3. Dethlefsen LA, Dewey WC (eds): Third International Symposium: Cancer Therapy by Hyperthermia, Drugs, and Radiation (Symposium held at Colorado State University, Fort Collins, CO, June 22–26, 1980). National Cancer Institute Monograph 61. Department of Health and Human Services, Public Health Service, National Institutes of Health, Bethesda, MD, 1982

4. Nussbaum GH (ed): Physical Aspects of Hyperthermia. American Association of Physicists in Medicine, Medical Physics, Monograph No. 8. American Institute of Physics, New York, 1982

5. Hahn GM: Hyperthermia and Cancer. Plenum Press, New York, 1982

6. Storm KF (ed): Hyperthermia in Cancer Therapy. GK Hall Medical Publishers, Boston, 1982
7. Lele PP: Hyperthermia by ultrasound. p. 168. In Wizenberg MJ, Robinson JE (eds): Proceedings of the International Symposium of Cancer Therapy by Hyperthermia and Radiation, American College of Radiology, Washington, DC, April 28–30, 1975
8. Lele PP: Induction of deep, local hyperthermia by ultrasound and electromagnetic fields. Radiat Environ Biophys 17:205, 1980
9. Lele PP: An annular-focus ultrasonic lens for production of uniform hyperthermia in cancer therapy. Ultrasound Med Biol 7:191, 1981
10. Lele PP: Local hyperthermia by ultrasound. p. 393. In Nussbaum GH (ed): Physical Aspects of Hyperthermia. Medical Physics Monograph No. 8, American Association of Physicists in Medicine. American Institute of Physics, New York, 1982
11. Lele PP: Physical aspects and clinical studies with ultrasonic hyperthermia. p. 333. In Storm FK (ed): Hyperthermia in Cancer Therapy. GK Hall Medical Publishers, Boston, 1983
12. Lele PP, Parker KJ: Temperature distributions in tissues during local hyperthermia by stationary or steered beams of unfocused or focused ultrasound. Br J Cancer, 45: suppl. V, 108–121, 1982
13. Goss SA, Frizzell LA, Dunn F (1979): Ultrasonic absorption and attenuation in mammalian tissues. Ultrasound Med Biol 5:181, 1979
14. Parker KJ, Lele PP: "The thermal pulse-decay method for determining ultrasound absorption coefficients. p. 754. In McAvoy BR (ed): Ultrasonics Symposium. IEEE Press. Piscataway, NJ, 1982
15. Lele PP: Thresholds and mechanisms of ultrasonic damage to 'organized animal' tissues. p. 224. In Hazzard DG, Litz ML (eds): Symposium on Biological Effects and Characterizations of Ultrasound Sources. Proceedings of a Conference held in Rockville, MD, June 2–3, 1977. Department of Health, Education and Welfare Publication (FDA) 78–8048. Rockville, MD, 1977
16. Marmor JB, Pounds D, Postic TB, Hahn GM: Treatment of superficial human neoplasms by local hyperthermia induced by ultrasound. Cancer 43:188, 1979
17. Marmor JB, Pounds D, Hahn N, Hahn GM: Treating spontaneous tumors in dogs and cats by ultrasound-induced hyperthermia. Int J Radiat Oncol Biol Phys 4:967, 1978
18. Babayan RK, Lele PP, Krane RJ: Thermochemotherapy of renal adenocarcinoma in Wistar-Lewis rats. p. 142. In Proceedings of 77th Annual Meeting of American Urological Association, May 16–20, 1982. Bartle Hall and Radisson-Muehlebach, Kansas City, MO, 1982
19. Lele PP: Temperature-duration thresholds for irreversible histologic and/or ultrastructural damage to normal mammalian tissues and tumors *in vivo*. p. 6. In Broerse JJ, Barendsen GW, Kal HB, et al (eds): Tumor Biology and Therapy, Proceedings 7th International Congress of Radiation Research, Amsterdam, July 3–8, 1983. Martinus Nijhoff, The Hague, 1983
20. Lele PP: Local hyperthermia for advanced squamous carcinoma of the head and neck: an attractive candidate for combined modality studies. In Wolf GT (ed): Head and Neck Cancer, Advances in Treatment. Martinus Nijhoff, Hingham, MA (in press)

13 Surgical Applications of Ultrasound

PETER N.T. WELLS

The applications of ultrasound to surgery can broadly be considered in two different classes, depending on the ultrasonic frequency. First, high-frequency ultrasound, in the frequency range 1–10 MHz, is used to deposit energy in localized soft-tissue sites. The ultrasound may be focused, and the lesion may be beneath intervening tissue which remains undamaged. The mechanism which produces the desired damage or biological change is always at least partly thermal, although cavitation and perhaps other effects may have a role. The second class of surgical applications exploits the direct effects of mechanical vibrations in the ultrasonic frequency range 20–50 kHz. Usually, an instrument with a hard vibrating tip is used to cut or shatter hard tissues or calculi, or to cut or emulsify soft tissues. In specialized applications, the heat accompanying the process may contribute to the surgical objective. Low-frequency vibrations in the form of focused shock waves can also be applied transcutaneously to disintegrate calculi without damaging the surrounding tissues.

Strictly speaking, the word "surgery" means the treatment of injuries or diseases by manual operation. While many of the applications of ultrasound described in this chapter fall within this definition, some of the procedures use ultrasound to induce effects which are intended to have smaller risk/benefit ratios than the conventional surgical cutting operations which they aim to replace.

SURGICAL APPLICATIONS OF HIGH-FREQUENCY ULTRASOUND

Neurosurgery

The possibility that ultrasound might be used for brain surgery was first tried 40 years ago. Lynn and Putnam[1] exposed the brains of 3 dogs, 30 cats, and 4 monkeys to a strongly focused beam of 835 kHz ultrasound. The results, which were disastrous for the animals, were not helpful scientifically because the exposure conditions were not recorded. Moreover, the investigators did not realise the importance of bone as an attenuator. They wrote that "in contrast to the cats and dogs, the monkeys were especially satisfactory experimental animals because of the almost complete lack of radiation-absorbing muscle tissue over the skull areas."

Ten years later, in 1954, Lindstrom[2] treated 20 patients, 16 of whom had intractable pain due to metastatic tumors, with unfocused ultrasound as a substitute for lobotomy. The intensity used was 7 W/cm², applied for 4–14 minutes through a suitable hole in the skull. The postoperative course in every case was apparently satisfactory and without complication. Similar equipment was later used, following successful experiments with induced epilepsy in cats, to treat three human patients; the frequencies of their attacks were usefully reduced.[3]

In principle, high-frequency ultrasonic surgery has two main advantages over conventional techniques involving cutting. Firstly, the ultrasound can be deposited, by means of appropriately designed applicators, in such a way that selected deep structures are modified or destroyed while intervening tissue remains undamaged. Secondly, the tissue modification is accomplished without damage to blood vessels, so there is no hemorrhage.

These two advantages are realized most elegantly by the use of a focused ultrasonic beam. In a lossless medium, such a beam has maximum intensity—and hence, maximum surgical "efficacy"—in the focal volume. In an attenuating medium such as biological soft tissue the gain in intensity toward the focus is to some extent offset by the loss of ultrasonic energy in the intervening medium, which itself increases with frequency. Superimposed on these effects is the cooling due to conduction and blood flow. Consequently, for any particular depth of penetration, it is necessary to compromise between beam convergence angle, lesion geometry, ultrasonic frequency, and exposure time. A typical arrangement for focused ultrasonic human neurosurgery (Fig 13.1) uses a flat disc transducer, with a resonant frequency of around 1 MHz, and a diameter of about 10 cm, mounted with an air backing and a concave plastic lens arranged to focus the beam through a conical angle of about 50°. The transducer may be operated at its fundamental frequency of 1 MHz, or at its third harmonic frequency of 3 MHz. When arranged for brain lesion production, the exposure conditions at the focus[4, 5] are usually chosen to lie somewhere between 20 kW/cm² for 300 μsec and 200 W/cm² (spatial-peak intensities measured in situ) for 10 seconds. At the highest intensities, the process of lesion production appears to include a contribution from a direct mechanical effect (perhaps cavitation), whereas below about 200 W/cm², ultrasonic lesions seem to be of purely thermal origin.

The advantages of ultrasonic neurosurgery[6] include: the ability to produce permanent lesions of any shape, size, and orientation at any site, without disrupting the intervening tissue; the ability to produce temporary or permanent changes in basic functions, by appropriate choice of dosage; the maintenance of the intact vascular system in cerebral regions where all neuronal elements are destroyed; the selective damage of white matter without involving grey matter; and the low incidence of morbidity and mortality. In attempts to exploit these advantages, ultrasonic neurosurgery has been used in the treatment of the following clinical conditions:

Parkinsons' Disease

The rationale of the direct methods is that the symptoms of hyperkinesia and hypertonus can be alleviated by interrupting the appropriate neural pathways within the brain. Assuming that these pathways can be identified, focused ultrasound is an ideal candidate for the trackless placement of the necessary lesions. In one series,[7] 15 operations were carried out on 12 patients, with the ansa lenticularis and the substantia nigra as targets. Following preliminary craniotomies, the ultrasonic irradiations were carried out under local anesthesia so that the functional modification could be assessed.

Diseases Controlled by the Pituitary Gland

The metastases of patients with breast or prostate cancer can sometimes be controlled by hypophysectomy resulting in the withdrawal of pituitary stimuli to the adrenal glands and the ovaries or the testes. The progress of other diseases, for example, diabetic retinopathy, is also controlled by the pituitary. Interruption of the pituitary function can be accomplished by surgery, but none of the customary surgical approaches is ideal. Alternatively, the pituitary can be ablated by ionizing radiation (external beams or implanted sources), stereotactic cryosurgery, or ultrasound. Using an approach similar to that for the treatment of Parkinson's disease with focused ultrasound, five patients with breast cancer have been treated but without significantly favorable alterations in malignant growth patterns; moreover, the postoperative complications were seriously debilitating.[8] It is interesting to note that one of the postoperative complications of conventional surgical removal of the pituitary gland by the trans-ethmoid-sphenoid route is that of the leakage of cerebrospinal fluid, and that there have been several attempts to ablate the pituitary by applying ultrasound using this approach but through the intact dura.[9, 10] There seems to be no evidence, however, that an adequate exposure can be applied in this way to destroy the whole gland, or that ultrasound can be used selectively to destroy cells of a specific type.

Intractable Pain

In the spinal cord, nerve fibers conducting pain impulses cross in the posterior commissure, whereas those conducting sensory and motor impulses do not. This opens up the possibility that intractable pelvic pain such as that due to malignant disease might be alleviated by commissurotomy. Conventional surgery is usually followed by paralysis due to interruption of the posterior spinal artery. It has been shown in experiments on cats, however, that focused ultrasound can be used to destroy nerve fibers in the posterior commissure and

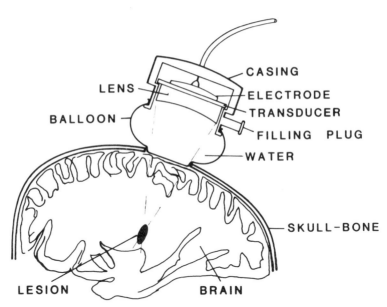

FIG. 13.1 Typical arrangement for focused ultrasonic neurosurgery. In this example, the balloon is filled with water to couple the ultrasound from the lens to the dura which is left intact over the brain.

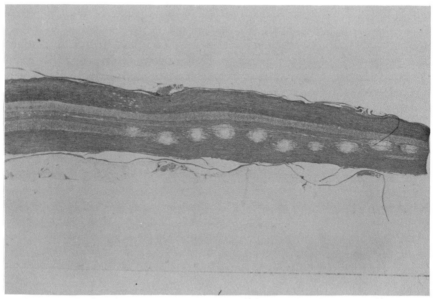

FIG. 13.2 Lesions placed in the posterior commissure of the spinal cord by means of focused ultrasound. The lesions, which have the typical "island and moat" appearance, are placed at intervals of about 2 mm. The specimen was removed after death from a patient whose ultrasonic treatment had been designed to alleviate intractable pain. (Courtesy of Dr. B. Browell, Mr. H. B. Griffith and Dr. M. Halliwell.)

that lesions can be placed side by side over a segment of adequate length to destroy the pain-conducting fibers without interfering with the sensory and motor functions.[11] Despite the fact that laminectomy is required to remove the bone overlying the spinal cord, operations on humans have been carried out using a 3-MHz system and a spatial peak intensity of about 150 W/cm^2 in situ producing spherical lesions (Fig. 13.2) of about 1 mm diameter with an exposure of 2 seconds. In some patients the results appear to have been encouraging, but the numbers are too small to be conclusive.[12]

Focused ultrasonic surgery has a limited but important place in the study of neuroanatomic pathways, and in the treatment of experimentally induced abnormalities. For example, it has been shown that the corpus callosum can be severed to obtain split-brain rats for behavioral investigations.[13]

The elegant and classical work which led to the development of focused-beam techniques for brain surgery was stimulated by the gloomy prospects faced by patients whose only alternative treatment was conventional surgery. Since that time, advances in pharmaceuticals and changing fashions in medicine have largely eliminated the demand for the ultrasonic approach, except perhaps in the case of commissurotomy where the potential advantages are significant but not yet widely recognized. It is for these reasons that the contemporary applications of ultrasonic neurosurgery are limited to the laboratories of the experimental neuroanatomists and neurophysiologists. One of the principal discouragements to the development of focused ultrasonic neurosurgery has been the presumption that it is necessary to remove bone to provide access to the brain. It has recently been demonstrated, however, that predictable and reproducible lesioning is possible through the intact skull by lowering the ultrasonic frequency to 500 kHz.[14] Perhaps this may lead to a resurgence of interest in the techniques.

Vestibular Surgery

Ultrasonic irradiation of the vestibular end organ for the treatment of Meniere's disease was first reported by Krejci in 1952.[15] He applied ultrasound transcutaneously to the temporal bone, and his patient was apparently cured with his hearing improved.

Meniere's disease, which results in attacks of vertigo and tinnitus, seems to be due to abnormally raised endolymphatic pressure in the inner ear. The attacks often seem to be psychologically triggered; it is often suggested that Krejci's treatment triggered the psychological cure of his patient. In any event, it is clear that only an insignificant fraction of ultrasound could have reached the vestibular apparatus after traveling through the temporal bone. It was left to Arslan[16] to pioneer the technique of surgically exposing the lateral semicircular canal for the direct application of ultrasound. Arslan's idea was taken up and refined by several independent groups of investigators. The objective of these investigations was to apply the ultrasound to the vestibular end organ while avoiding irradiating the cochlea and damaging the nearby facial nerve with excessive heat.

A technique which is still in routine use employs a probe with a 3-MHz transducer of 5 mm diameter mounted at the larger end of a small hollow metal funnel which concentrates the ultrasound along a short tube, 2 mm in diameter. The ultrasound is propagated through physiologic saline solution which fills the cone and tube and which flows continuously to cool the transducer and the prepared surface of the bone (Fig. 13.3).[17] Thermocouple experiments with postmortem temporal bones, prepared as for ultrasonic irradiation of the lateral semicircular canal, indicated that the temperature of the facial nerve canal does not exceed 48°C provided that the ultrasonic power is kept below 700 mW. This seems to be a safe temperature; higher temperatures are associated with the risk of facial nerve paralysis, either immediately or within a few days as a result of edema.

The level of surgical skill necessary for the exposure of the lateral semicircular canal for ultrasonic irradiation by the transtemporal approach is considerable, as it is necessary for the bone to be burred down to about 0.5 mm thickness, to ensure good transmission of ultrasound and the establishment of the appropriate thermal distribution, but the bone must not be fractured or perilymph may escape and air bubbles may form. Because of this difficulty, the technique of direct application of ultrasound through the middle ear by means of a 1.5-mm-diameter, 3.5-MHz transducer placed in the round window was developed.[18] The distance from the facial nerve is greater than that from the lateral semicircular canal, and so this approach is inherently safer. Moreover, good results are apparently obtained with a power of up to only 100 mW. This corresponds to a spatial-average temporal-average (SATA) intensity, I_t, equal to 5.7 W/cm^2 (See Chapter 2).

The justification for the complexity of the ultrasonic treatment is that it offers the likelihood that the patient will retain his hearing besides being cured of the symptoms of Meniere's disease. Alternative surgical techniques either result in total destruction of the vestibular end organ (including the cochlea), or involve the technically very difficult division of the vestibular branch of the eighth nerve. The mechanism by which ultrasound achieves its effect, however, is not clear. The results of animal experiments[19] suggest that both heat and some direct effect of ultrasound are involved. It may be that the treatment locally interrupts the integrity of the membrane that forms the barrier between the endolymphatic and perilymphatic compartments, thus relieving the endolymphatic pressure. The associated change in the ionic balance of the endolymph might be confined to the neighborhood of the site of the lesions, leading to histologic changes in the vestibular apparatus but not in the cochlea.

Other Applications

Treatment of Laryngeal Papillomatosis

Benign epithelial tumors of the larynx are rare, but when multiple papillomata occur they can obstruct the airway. Surgical excision is not often satisfactory, because the condition usually recurs. Following this surgery, however, direct

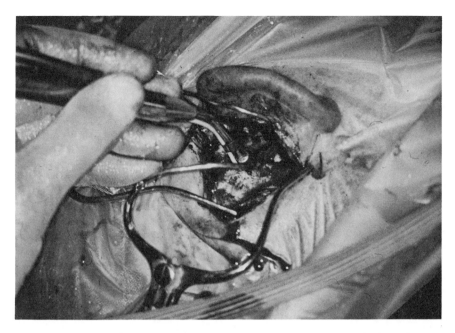

FIG. 13.3 Treatment of Meniere's disease by ultrasonic irradiation of the lateral semicircular canal. The end of the probe carries a 3-MHz ultrasonic transducer with a diameter of 5 mm and the beam is guided through a liquid-filled tube with a diameter of 2 mm in contact with the thin surgically prepared bone layer over the semicircular canal. The exposure time is about 20 minutes at a power of 700 mW. (Courtesy of Mr. J. A. James.)

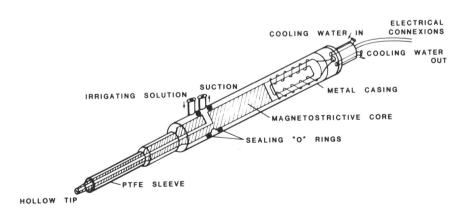

FIG. 13.4 Diagram showing the construction of an ultrasonic surgical aspirator. The hollow tip of the instrument has an outside diameter of about 2 mm, and only the part exposed beyond the plastic [polytetrafluoroethylene (PTFE)] sleeve is active. The emulsified tissue is removed by suction aspiration of the irrigating saline solution.

application of ultrasound may eliminate the disease possibly by thermal sterilization of a causative virus. A typical treatment is a 5-minute application of 9-MHz ultrasound from a 5-mm transducer delivering 150 mW.[20] In children, the treatment may need to be repeated several times at intervals of three months.

Applications in Ophthalmology

The ability of ultrasound to induce several potentially important changes in the eye is presently being studied. Focused 10-MHz ultrasound has been used to produce lesions on the retina and choroid in the rabbit eye.[21, 22] Ultimately it may be possible to place therapeutic lesions at sites made inaccessible to laser surgery by overlying opaque tissue or blood, or at sites that do not absorb light. Another possible ophthalmic application is for the treatment of myopia. It has been reported[23] that irradiation of the whole intact globe with 850 kHz ultrasound at intensities of up to 1.5 W/cm² produces an average reduction of 1.0 D in refraction in patients under 20 years of age. The suggested mechanism is that the ultrasound may affect the ciliary muscle.

Contraception and Termination of Pregnancy

Following experiments on male cats, dogs, and monkeys, in which spermatogenesis was suppressed by transcutaneous irradiation of the testes for 10–15 minutes with 1.1 MHz ultrasound at intensities of 1–2 W/cm⁻² , encouraging results were obtained in humans.[24] The treatment was painless and there were no side effects reported. Whether or not the method could be used for everyday contraception remains to be determined. Another proposal which still has to be tested is that pregnancy might be terminated by the delivery of similar or higher intensities of ultrasound, either focused transabdominally or delivered through the cervix.[25]

SURGICAL APPLICATION OF LOW-FREQUENCY ULTRASOUND

Cataract Surgery

Although congenital cataracts can be aspirated through an incision of only 2–3 mm in length, senile cataracts require an incision extending through half the capsule, and having a length of 10–15 mm.

The application of high-amplitude (approximately 300 μm peak-to-peak tip displacement), low-frequency (23-kHz) ultrasound can emulsify a senile cataract in situ, and the incision required to introduce the working tip of the instrument (Fig. 13.4)[26] is only 2–3 mm long. The advantages of the operation, in comparison with conventional surgery, is that the patient can be discharged from hospital after only a couple of days, the procedure is safe, and the optical result is free from astigmatism.[27]

Soft Tissue Surgery

An ultrasonic surgical aspirator has been developed from the instrument used for phacoemulsification and described in the previous section. Application of the tip of the instrument to soft tissue results, at high amplitude, in emulsification and removal of the material within a 1- to 2-mm radius.[28] Tissues with high water content are most readily fragmented, but care is needed to avoid puncturing blood vessels despite their high collagen content.

There are three modes of action for the ultrasonic surgical aspirator. At low amplitude, tissues and particularly blood vessels can be dissected; at medium amplitude, cutting is possible; and at high amplitude tissues can be aspirated. The technique is relatively bloodless. Encouraging results have been obtained in brain tumor excision[29] and in total pancreatectomy, partial hepatectomy, tongue resection, and rectal cancer surgery.[30]

In vascular surgery, the ultrasonic aspiration can be used to remove soft thrombus.[31] It can also be used for endarterectomy, where it has the advantage over conventional spatula dissection that the free residual edge of the intima can be made level.[32]

Calculus Disintegration

Endoscopic ultrasonic disintegration of renal, bladder, and urethral stones is emerging as an attractive alternative to open surgery. A rigid metal rod of about 3 mm diameter is used to apply ultrasound in the frequency range 22–30 kHz directly to the calculus under endoscopic vision.[33,34] The excursion amplitude of the tip is too small to damage soft tissue into which it may come into contact. The stone is methodically broken into fragments small enough to be removed by aspiration through a tube mounted beside the endoscope, or to be passed naturally.

As an alternative to percutaneous ultrasonic disintegration, a machine has been developed which can disintegrate renal stones by focused shock waves applied transcutaneously under x-ray imaging control.[35] The shock waves are produced by an underwater spark generator mounted at the near focus of an ellipsoid; the stone is positioned at the far focus. A course of treatment may last 20–30 minutes during which time 500–1,000 shocks are applied to break the stone into fragments small enough to be passed without cholic.

Dental Applications

Instruments like the ultrasonic surgical aspirator described earlier in this section are again gaining popularity in dentistry, after the static period since the 1960s when their potential was first discussed.[36] In comparison with rotating tools, ultrasonic instruments are popular with patients. The applications for which they are appropriate include root canal reaming,[37] cleaning and calculus removal, gingevectomy, orthodontic filing, amalgam packing, and gold foil manipulation.

Bone Cutting and Welding

The use of ultrasound for cutting bone has several potential advantages over conventional methods. The instrument consists of a fine-toothed saw mounted at the end of an ultrasonic driver operating at a frequency of 20–50 kHz, with a peak-to-peak displacement amplitude of 50–80 μm. The cutting speed is about the same as that of a regular saw, but much less pressure is needed.[38] It is easier to keep to the desired osteotomy line, and the cut surface, although rough, is free from microfractures.

In bone welding, the penetration rate and chemical curing of cyanoacrylate adhesive are both significantly accelerated by the application of ultrasound under similar conditions to that used for bone cutting.[39] Apertures can be filled with bone chips in cyanoacrylate. Following the welding process, natural bone regeneration occurs; live cells eventually cover or penetrate the adhesive and the filler material becomes perfused with blood.

REFERENCES

1. Lynn JG, Putnam TJ: Histology of cerebral lesions produced by ultrasound. Am J Pathol 20:637, 1944
2. Lindstrom PA: Prefrontal ultrasonic irradiation—a substitute for lobotomy. Arch Neurol Psychiatr 72:399, 1954
3. Lindstrom PA, Beck EC: Suppression of epileptic movements in the presence of grand mal seizure discharges. J Neurosurg 20:97, 1963
4. Fry FJ, Kossoff G, Eggleton RC, Dunn F: Threshold ultrasonic dosages for structural changes in the mammalian brain. J Acoust Soc Am 48:1413, 1970
5. Pond JB: The role of heat in the production of ultrasonic focal lesions. J Acoust Soc Am 47:1607, 1970
6. Meyers R, Fry FJ, Fry WJ, et al: Determination of topologic human brain representations and modifications of signs and symptoms of some neurologic disorders by the use of high level ultrasound. Neurology 10:271, 1960
7. Meyers R, Fry WJ, Fry FJ, et al: Early experiences with ultrasonic irradiation of the pallidofugal and nigral complexes in hyperkinetic and hypertonic disorders. J Neurosurg 16:32, 1959
8. Hickey RC, Fry WJ, Meyers R, et al: Human pituitary irradiation with focused ultrasound. Arch Surg 83:620, 1961
9. Arslan M. Ultrasound hypophysectomy. J Laryngol Otol 20:73, 1964
10. Giancarlo HR, Mattuci KF: Effect of ultrasonic hypophysectomy on diabetic retinopathy. Laryngoscope 81:452, 1971
11. Richards DE, Typer CF, Shealey CN: Focused ultrasonic spinal commissurotomy: experimental evaluation. J Neurosurg 24:701, 1966
12. Griffith HB, Brownell JB, Halliwell M, Wells PN: Arterial damage by trackless lesions in the spinal cord made by focused ultrasound. Br J Surg 60:899, 1973
13. Lee AJ, Taberner PV, Halliwell M: Severing the corpus callosum in rats using ultrasound: theoretical and experimental correlations. J Acoust Soc Am 66:1292, 1979

14. Fry FJ, Goss SA: Further studies of the transkull transmission of an intense focused ultrasonic beam: lesion production at 500 kHz. Ultrasound Med Biol 6:33, 1980

15. Krejci F: Experimentelle Grundlagen einer extralabyrinthären chirurgischen Behandlungsmethode der Ménièreschen Erkankung. Pract Otorhinolarnygol 14:18, 1952

16. Arslan M: Ultrasonic surgery of the labyrinth in patients with Meniere's syndrome. Sci Med Ital 7:301, 1958

17. James JA, Dalton GA, Hadley KJ, et al: A new 3-megacycle generator for destruction of the vestibular end organ. Acta Otolaryngol 56:148, 1963

18. Kossoff G, Wadsworth JR, Dudley PF: The round window ultrasonic technique for treatment of Meniere's disease. Arch Otolaryngol 86:535, 1967

19. Barnett SB: The influence of ultrasound and temperature on the cochlear microphonic response following a round window irradiation. Acta Octolaryngol 90:32, 1980

20. White A, Halliwell M, Fairman HD: Ultrasonic treatment of laryngeal papillomata. J Laryngol Otol 88:249, 1974

21. Lizzi FL, Coleman DJ, Driller J, et al: Experimental, ultrasonically induced lesions in the retina, choroid and sclera. Invest Ophthalmol 17:350, 1978

22. Lizzi FL, Coleman DJ, Driller J, et al: Effects of pulsed ultrasound on ocular tissue. Ultrasound Med Biol 7:245, 1981

23. Greguss P, Bertenyi A: A critical analysis of ultrasonic therapy. Ultrasonics 14:81, 1976

24. Fahim MS, Fahim Z, Harman J, et al: Ultrasound as a new method of male contraception. Fertil Steril 28:823, 1977

25. Sikov MR: Ultrasound: its potential use for the termination of pregnancy. Contraception 8:429, 1973

26. Kelman CD: Phaco-emulsification and aspiration. Am J Ophthalmol 67:464, 1969

27. Arnott E: The ultrasonic technique for cataract removal. Trans Ophthalmol Soc UK 93:33, 1973

28. Hodgson WJB: Ultrasonic surgery. Ann R Coll Surg Engl 62:459, 1980

29. Flamm ES, Ransohoff J, Wunchinich D, Broadwin A: Preliminary experience with ultrasonic aspiration in neurosurgery. Neurosurgery 2:240, 1978

30. Hodgson WJB, Bakare S, Harrington E, et al: General surgical evaluation of a powered device operating at ultrasonic frequencies. Mt Sinai J Med 46:99, 1979

31. Stumpff U, Pohlman R, Trübestein G: A new method to cure thrombi by ultrasonic cavitation. p. 273. In Ultrasonics International 1975. IPC Science and Technology Press, Guildford, England, 1975

32. Finkelstein JL, Hodgson WJB, McElhinney AJ, Aufses AH: Preliminary feasibility studies using an ultrasonic device for endarterectomy. Mt Sinai J Med 46:107, 1979

33. Alken P, Hutschenreiter G, Gunther R, Marberger M: Percutaneous stone manipulation. J Urol 125:463, 1981

34. El Fahiq S, Wallace DM: Ultrasonic lithotriptor for urethral and bladder stones. Br J Urol 50:255, 1978

35. Chaussy C, Schmiedt E, Jocham D, et al: First clinical experience with extracorporeally induced destruction of kidney stones by shock waves. J Urol 127:417, 1982

36. Balamuth L: The application of ultrasonic energy in the dental field. p. 194. In Brown B, Gordon D (eds): Ultrasonic Techniques in Biology and Medicine. Iliffe, London, 1967

37. Cunningham WJ, Martin H, Forrest WR: Evaluation of root canal débridement by the endosonic ultrasonic synergistic system. Oral Surg 53:401, 1982

38. Aro H, Kallioniemi H, Aho AJ, Kellokumpi-Lehtinen P: Ultrasonic device in bone cutting. Acta Orthop Scand 52:5, 1981

39. Volkov MV, Shepeleva IS: The use of ultrasonic instrumentation for the transection and uniting of bone tissue in orthopedic surgery. Reconstr Surg Traumatol 14:147, 1974

14 Standards and Guidelines for Medical Ultrasound

MARVIN C. ZISKIN
WESLEY L. NYBORG

From the information presented in previous chapters of this volume, little basis is given for expecting damage to patients from customary applications of ultrasonic therapy, and even less basis for harm from accepted practice of diagnostic ultrasound. However, it is recognized that adverse effects which are delayed, or which occur infrequently, cannot be ruled out. Also, there is no doubt that harm could result if ultrasound was applied unwisely. In the interests of caution and the public welfare, various professional groups and governmental agencies have adopted or proposed standards and guidelines for manufacturers and users of medical ultrasound equipment.

This chapter is divided into two parts. Part A is a factual account of the activities and recommendations by private organizations, as well as guidelines and regulations issued by governmental agencies, pertaining to equipment for medical ultrasound and to its clinical use. Here editorial comments and value judgments have been minimized. Part B, on the other hand, presents personal opinions and advice from respected individual colleagues.

PART A: ORGANIZATIONAL ACTIVITIES AND RECOMMENDATIONS

Standards for Equipment

To promote good medical practice in the use of ultrasonic equipment, it is necessary to employ uniform nomenclature and to follow standard procedures for assessing equipment performance. The American Institute of Ultrasound in Medicine (AIUM) has adopted and published a number of performance standards for diagnostic equipment,[1, 2] as well as a compilation of approved nomenclature.[3] Included in the latter are definitions of *frequency, acoustic power,* various indices of *acoustic intensity,* and other parameters needed for specifying the output of medical ultrasound equipment. These parameters are discussed and used in Chapter 2 and Appendix A of this volume.

A number of countries have adopted governmental standards requiring acoustic output specifications for therapeutic and/or diagnostic ultrasound devices. Since 1978 the US Food and Drug Administration (FDA) has enforced performance standards for ultrasonic therapy equipment; these require manufacturers to provide acoustic intensity specifications and other output data with their equipment.[4] Standards adopted by Canada in 1981 are similar, except that these include a regulation that the spatial-average temporal-peak (SATP) intensity (measured at the transducer) shall not exceed 3 W/cm². [5, 6]

Such Federal requirements do not exist in the United States or Canada for diagnostic equipment, although in 1979 the FDA published a Notice of Intent to Propose Rules and Develop Recommendations for Diagnostic Ultrasound Equipment.[7] A purpose in publishing the "Notice of Intent" was to encourage nongovernmental groups to propose standards; these would be accepted on a voluntary basis, at least until such time as a mandatory federal standard might seem appropriate. A response was made by the National Electrical Manufacturers Association (NEMA) jointly with the AIUM in developing a voluntary standard which was published in 1982.[8] In the AIUM-NEMA standard, parameters are defined which are to be used by manufacturers in specifying the acoustic output of diagnostic ultrasound equipment. Examples of these specifications are given in Appendix A.

The intensities defined in Chapter 2 are called *exposure parameters* since they are selected as indicators of the ultrasonic exposure received by a patient in a therapy treatment or in a diagnostic examination. These parameters, together with the time of exposure are believed to be measures of the extent to which the ultrasound exposure will affect, or might affect, the patient. For the therapist using ultrasound it is important to know these parameters, and adjust them so that the desired improvement in the patient can be achieved without unwanted side effects. For the physician or sonographer using diagnostic ultrasound, knowledge of these parameters may allow choices to be made for getting desired diagnostic information while minimizing the patient exposure.

Specifications on the exposure parameters are provided for all ultrasonic therapy equipment, as required by law. For diagnostic equipment these specifications are made public only when the manufacturer chooses to do so. In an effort to encourage publication of the data for diagnostic equipment, the AIUM awards Certificates of Commendation to manufacturers who make reliable information on exposure parameters conveniently available to prospective customers.[9] The data given in Table A.1 of Appendix A are from firms who have received this Commendation.

Guidelines for Equipment

In addition to the governmental regulations which have been adopted for commercial medical ultrasound equipment, there are weaker constraints which exist through guidelines and recommendations from agencies, committees, and groups.

For example, the FDA,[7] the Canadian Environmental Health Directorate (EHD),[6] the AIUM,[10] the National Council of Radiation Protection and Measurements (NCRP),[11] and the World Health Organization[12] all urge that output data for diagnostic equipment be made available to users. Thus, it is widely agreed that the medical community should be well provided with information on this aspect of equipment performance. It is hoped that physicians and sonographers will be able to use these data, along with other information, in making decisions on equipment and procedures.

Advice has varied as to any upper limits applicable to output intensities of diagnostic equipment. The FDA has suggested that an intensity I_t of 10 mW/cm² would be a reasonable upper limit for pulse-echo devices, and has posed the question of whether a spatial-peak temporal-average (SPTA) intensity of 100 mW/cm² should be imposed or recommended as a general upper limit for diagnostic devices. Several industrial standards have been established by the Japanese Standards Association, including a requirement for fetal Doppler equipment that the intensity I_t should not exceed 10 mW/cm².[12] The EHD urges manufacturers to "make every endeavor to design and construct equipment so that it functions at SATA intensities of less than 100 mW/cm²."[6] The World Health Organization, Regional Office for Europe,[13] chose not to recommend an upper limit but observed that "many diagnostic procedures can be carried out entirely satisfactorily under conditions such that the patient is exposed to a relatively low beam intensity, such as 100 W/m² temporal-spatial average, or less." (100 W/m² = 10 mW/cm².) In the AIUM-NEMA Standard are two general guidelines for diagnostic ultrasound equipment. These were endorsed (with a minor change of wording) by the NCRP[11] in the following form:

1. Ultrasound equipment should be designed so the maximum levels of the various intensities which the equipment can produce are as low as practicable for the anticipated uses of the equipment.

2. Where such flexibility is consistent with reasonable cost and performance of the system, operators should be able to adjust controls to use the minimum acoustic intensity required to image the desired organs on each patient.

Guidelines for Medical Practice

Considerably more detailed advice has been given for the clinical use of ultrasound in therapy than in diagnosis. This is reasonable since therapeutic applications involve use of higher intensities, and physiologic changes are deliberately sought. According to recommendations from the EHD[6] and the NCRP,[11] therapists are urged to use intensities and exposure times that are no more than are needed to achieve the desired clinical benefit. The operator should be alert to any sign of distress of the patient; if pain is experienced, the applicator should be moved more rapidly and/or the intensity should be decreased. Pregnant patients should never receive ultrasound therapy in such a way that exposure of the fetus is likely. Also other specific precautions are given, such as to avoid exposing epiphyseal lines of bones in children.

For users of diagnostic ultrasound the most specific recommendation is probably one from the NCRP:[11]

> Routine ultrasound examination of the human fetus should not be performed under exposure conditions where a significant temperature elevation might be expected.

In discussing the above recommendation it is stated that "since normal diurnal temperature variation exceeds 1°C, temperature elevations less than 1°C are usually not considered significant." It is also judged to be "highly unlikely that in clinical practice using a current commercially available diagnostic unit the intra-uterine temperature would be raised as much as 1°C." The NCRP recommendation cited above is made in reference to the possibility of abnormal exposures, in which equipment of unusually high output is used for an extended time.

Other advice to users of diagnostic ultrasound has been of a fairly general nature, recognizing the responsibility of the physician to make informed medical decisions, weighing expected benefits against potential risks. Important to the process of making such decisions is an awareness of equipment parameters and their significance. Typical of advice to users is a recommendation by the NCRP:[11]

> They should strive to obtain the most medically significant information while producing the least ultrasonic exposure to the patient. By the latter is meant, specifically, that dwell times and total exposure times should be minimized and, where adjustable, intensities should also be minimized.

In the last sentence above, the phrase "dwell time" refers to the time during which the ultrasound beam is directed to a particular region of a patient's body, while "exposure time" refers to the total time of the examination.

Related to this is the advice from the AIUM to "give serious consideration to intensity data when comparing various instruments"; at the same time the AIUM warns against an oversimplistic view on the role of "intensity." Relatively high intensities may sometimes be needed in order to obtain important diagnostic information.[10] The necessity for judgment in the choice of intensity (when a choice is available) is expressed by the World Health Organization in these terms: "other factors (e.g., system noise level, bandwith) being equal, there is a direct relationship between the diagnostic information obtainable by a particular technique and the level of primary ultrasound energy directed into a patient."[13]

Because of concern over safety of diagnostic ultrasound imaging in pregnancy, and concern over whether all that which is performed is actually necessary or appropriate, several of the institutes of the National Institutes of Health together with the National Center for Devices and Radiological Health sponsored a Consensus Development Conference on this topic. This conference brought together scientists, health professionals, consumers, and the public to hear and comment upon a draft report proposed by a panel of experts. The following questions were addressed:

What types of ultrasound scanning are currently used in obstetric practice? How extensive is this use? What is known about the dose/exposure to the fetus and the mother from each type?

For what purposes is ultrasound now used in pregnancy? For each use what is the evidence that ultrasound improves patient management and/or outcome of pregnancy?

What are the theoretical risks of ultrasound to the fetus and the mother? What evidence exists from animal, tissue culture, and human studies on the actual extent of the risk?

Based on the available evidence, what are the appropriate indications for and limitations on the use of ultrasound in obstetrics today?

What further studies are needed of efficacy and safety of use of ultrasound in pregnancy?

Answers to the above questions were formulated based on the collective experience of the panel members, a year-long review of the scientific literature, and comments presented to the panel at the Consensus meeting. In addition, the panel made a number of specific recommendations.

Because of the lack of information on the amount of ultrasound a fetus is exposed to in the clinical setting, the panel recommended that the dwell time on the fetus and the type of machine be recorded for each imaging examination. They also recommended that the occurrence of exposure to Doppler devices be recorded.

With respect to medical indications, the panel listed 27 different situations in which ultrasound should be used in pregnancy or related conditions. However, because of a lack of statistical proof that routine screening improved pregnancy outcome, and because of an assumed hypothetical risk, the panel decided that routine screening in pregnancy could not be recommended at this time.

Given that the full potential of diagnostic ultrasound imaging is critically dependent on examiner training and experience, the panel recommended establishing minimum training requirements and uniform credentialing for physicians and sonographers performing ultrasound examinations.

In response to the final question, the panel recommended research in various areas, such as research into fundamental mechanisms leading to bioeffects, effects on embryonic and fetal development, and epidemiological studies of the efficacy of routine screening in pregnancy.

Finally, it is of interest to note that in May 1982, the New Jersey State Department of Health issued guidelines on the appropriate use of amniocentesis for genetic studies. The guidelines recommended that a pre-amniocentesis ultrasound examination be performed prior to every midtrimester amniocentesis and that the results should be made known to the physician performing the anmiocentesis. They further recommended that the amniocentesis ideally should be performed within an ultrasound facility.

PART B: PERSONAL VIEWPOINTS

Introduction

Editorial comments and value judgments were omitted from Part A in order to provide a presentation which is as factual and as unbiased as possible. This was certainly not because we feel that such value judgments are inappropriate. Quite the contrary; it is our guess that medical users are influenced at least as much by personal opinions and advice from respected individual colleagues as by the deliberations of committees and agencies.

Accordingly, we sent copies of Part A to selected leading ultrasound authorities and asked for their comments. We also provided the following list of questions to suggest specific subtopics which these scientists might wish to address in their responses:

Are standards and guidelines useful? If not, explain. If so, what should they deal with? How should they be generated? By whom?

Are present activities, guidelines, and so forth adequate to ensure safety in medical applications of ultrasound? If not, or if so, explain.

Do users of clinical ultrasound base decisions on equipment purchase, choice of diagnostic modality, choice of ultrasound exposure (intensity or duration) on safety considerations? Should they? Do you?

The only other direction was that their contributions would be circulated among all the respondents, and that following this they would have the opportunity to modify their comments. Interestingly, it turned out that there were very few requests for modification, and these were for very minor editorial changes.

Statements from Ultrasound Authorities

The following is the collection of invited comments from selected ultrasound authorities. The ordering is alphabetical by each author's last name.

●

Use of high temporal-peak intensities to achieve desired quality of information about tissues under the surface of the body is common practice in diagnostic ultrasound. At the present time, there is no direct evidence that these exposures cause any biological effects in human subjects. In the absence of evidence of hazard, it would be irrational to place arbitrary limits on the output of diagnostic devices in the name of "safety." On the other hand, we know from the theory of cavitation, from in vitro observations and from experiments on insect larvae that temporal-peak intensities that are much lower than the maximum values that are used in clinical practice can produce profound, deleterious effects if the physical conditions are just right.

Almost all medical procedures involve risk/benefit decisions. It is reasonable to expect that medical specialists who use diagnostic ultrasound will be informed so that they can make the same judgments regarding the value and potential risks of ultrasound that they would for any other clinical procedure. If transient cavitation were to occur, it could cause highly localized cell damage. From our knowledge of the cavitation process, we can say that if it does occur in the human body, it probably is rare. For this reason, it is extremely unlikely that effects, if they exist, would be revealed in epidemiologic studies. Therefore, decisions regarding human exposures will have to be made by extrapolation from observations made under controlled conditions in the laboratory. In almost any application of ultrasound except for prenatal care, the risk of such a rare, localized event would probably be acceptable. Knowledge available at the present time suggests that a very conservative approach to obstetrical practice would limit the temporal maximum intensities at the fetus to less than 10 W/cm² in routine examinations.

Edwin L. Carstensen, Ph.D.
Professor of Electrical Engineering
The University of Rochester
Rochester, New York

●

Any collaboration in science, whether between individuals or worldwide, calls for organization and agreement over the meanings and definitions of measured quantities and their units. Such agreement, moreover, needs to be intelligently based on the appropriateness of the quantities selected to describe the phenomena of interest—in the present case the biological changes consequent on exposure to ultrasonic fields.

One must aim eventually to ensure that all such agreements are acceptable internationally and, at this level, the main relevant organization is the International Electrotechnical Commission (IEC) which has recently completed preparation of a standard recommendation on medical ultrasonic fields (Characteristics and Calibration of Hydrophones for Operation in the Range 0.5 to 15 MHz). The IEC work has recognized the important (but often forgotten) fact that the current state of knowledge of ultrasound bioeffects is still a long way from identifying any single quantity (e.g., SPTA intensity, defined in Chapter 2) as being adequately predictive of consequent biological effect, in the sense that "absorbed dose" can be so used in ionizing radiation dosimetry. Thus IEC recommends that measurements should be made, as properly sampled functions of both space and time, of a fundamental field variable; acoustic pressure is chosen for the practical reason that hydrophones suitable for such measurement are either actually or potentially available.

Development of such techniques, and related recommendations is inevitably slow work but, until such time as they are properly established and accepted, and until the quality of related biological data is much improved, the many ad hoc standards and guidelines which have recently appeared (often more in response to political and administrative, rather than scientific, criteria), including some of those referred to in Part A above, must be regarded with healthy scepticism.

C.R. Hill, D.Sc.
Institute of Cancer Research
Royal Marsden Hospital
Sutton, Surrey, England

●

The average clinician, given a choice, would probably prefer to use a diagnostic ultrasound scanner that meets some "standard" of intensity that would be considered appropriate for current obstetrical practice, so that the issue of clinical safety would not arise. Many clinicians may already believe that such imaginary standards have already been applied to current equipment in the field. That there is a broad range of intensities produced by various instruments is a fact that will require education in order to place the issue of patient safety in perspective. In addition, as the context of ultrasound utilization in obstetrics continues to change and evolve, and as more ultrasound examinations are performed in everyday obstetric and gynecologic practice, the need for continued vigilance by organized and legitimate research and regulatory groups will grow.

Present guidelines are useful, but due to their technical nature and engineering orientation plus their voluntary nature, do not really have much impact on clinical practice. Machines are more often bought, not on the basis of safety considerations, but more on the issues of affordability, ease of use, and physical appearance, plus image quality. Manufacturers do respond to the desires of their prospective customers, however, and if clinicians were to begin to ask for this information when equipment purchase is being considered, then perhaps this would be perceived as a desirable marketing strategy and the intensities produced by various pieces of equipment would become more commonly known and understood. It would be interesting to survey users of ultrasound instrumentation currently in the field to ask them whether or not they know if their equipment is made by a manufacturer who has received the AIUM commendation award for divulging ultrasound intensity information.

Physician responsibility to understand the equipment he or she works with, together with heightened public awareness of the safety of ultrasound, will slowly force manufacturers and clinicians to make such information available in an easily understood format, and so incorporate a full discussion of acoustic intensities and power outputs into future marketing strategy. We clinicians can foster this approach by asking questions in this domain as often as possible of the salesman and company representatives with whom we come into contact. It will be noticed. This much we owe to the patients in our care.

Until such time as regulations regarding standards for equipment and for medical practice have some regulatory force and until such time as the issues of physician training and education have been more fully addressed, guidelines and recommendations of the various professional groups most closely involved with the development of diagnostic ultrasound can serve only as a means of increasing public and professional awareness of the issues that need to be resolved as the ultimate role of diagnostic ultrasound in obstetrics begins to emerge. Where we understand the issues, clear-cut guidelines and recommendations should be supported, and where there is ignorance it should be acknowledged. Where recommendations for further basic research to complement present knowledge can be made, they should be to the proper organizations, review committees, professional clinical groups, and probably most importantly the appropriate federal government agencies. Additionally, manufacturers can be expected to support some of the research and development work necessary to understand the biological effects of ultrasound, since part of their responsibility in marketing these devices is to insure the public safety as much as possible consistent with present knowledge as it develops.

Charles W. Hohler, M.D.
Director of Perinatology and
    Perinatal Ultrasound
St. Joseph's Hospital
    and Medical Center
Phoenix, Arizona

●

Clearly, guidelines regarding the safe use of any piece of medical equipment are essential. In medicine we must always be mindful of the dictum "do no harm." However, this axiom should not paralyze our activities and prevent progress. In ultrasound, as in every other field of medicine, a biological effect is not synonymous with an adverse or harmful effect. It is obvious that the risk/benefit ratio to any patient must be taken into account when any procedure is performed; but this does not imply that there should not be "any" risk to a patient. The concept of a risk-free society is untenable if life is to go and progress is to be made. Therefore, we must remain vigilant and continue independent investigations as to the hazards and ill effects of therapeutic and diagnostic ultrasound to the patient. In addition, we must keep in mind that microbe or animal models do not necessarily relate to human models. Finally, we must all strive to maintain a proper prospective of the use of ultrasound in humans.

Richard A. Meyer, M.D.
Division of Cardiology
Children's Hospital
Cincinnati, Ohio

●

I welcome the voluntary adoption of standards. The current cooperative effort between NEMA and AIUM offers a more rapid and flexible route towards standardization than the alternative by which standards are promulgated by government agencies. An epidemiologic study of the clinical safety of ultrasound has not been undertaken in this country, and I feel it is now too late to institute such a study. A major concern now should be the repeated insonation of ovaries stimulated to ovulate, since this may prove to be one of the most sensitive times for producing deleterious effects. The results of animal and plant experiments are of interest but whatever they show, careful observations in humans must eventually provide the most significant data of human risk.

Kenneth J. Taylor, M.D., Ph.D.
Professor of Diagnostic Imaging
Yale University School of Medicine
New Haven, Connecticut

•

In our complex society with the world becoming smaller each day with improved communications, it is essential that we have certain standards and guidelines to keep some semblance of uniformity and quality in our actions and functions of everyday life. Our government itself is an example at setting such norms. Medicine is certainly no exception. With the vast amount of knowledge accumulated today in the different areas of health care, it is impossible for each of us to know all the ramifications and intricate mechanisms involved in our diagnostic and therapeutic decision making. It is therefore essential that we have standards established so that we do not exceed boundaries and go beyond limits in such a way that harm may result.

Standards can be established only if adequate knowledge is available to determine the usefulness and safety of the procedure for which standards are being set. To overrun these boundaries and set standards where knowledge is not available may be detrimental. As an example, should we set standards for the power level of ultrasound and the exposure time to be used in examining the human fetus? Our knowledge of biological effects of ultrasound on the developing fetus is limited and although we recognize that at very high levels damage can result we have little knowledge of damage that may result within the wide range of low intensities. From the knowledge we have, we can set broad ranges of power levels and exposure time that may be used but they must not be too restrictive. Standards that are too rigid can be detrimental by limiting advancement as well as the good that may result from useful diagnostic testing. There is, as we have experienced in many areas, a middle ground in which progress can thrive and good can result.

We can set meaningful diagnostic, operator training, and competence standards and guidelines. We have sufficient experience and knowledge in those areas to make reasonable recommendations. These have been done, as evidenced by the guidelines proposed by the combined task force of AIUM, the American College of Obstetricians and Gynecologists (ACOG), and the American College of Radiology (ACR) on physician training, and the clinical standards demanded by all three organizations. A number of technical and procedural standards are also acceptable and proper such as labeling, equipment standardization, nomenclature, and so forth. Most of these standards are either in the process of being established or have already been established.

Horace E. Thompson, M.D.
Chairman, Department of
    Obstetrics and Gynecology
Louisiana State University
    School of Medicine
Shreveport, Louisiana

•

Voluntary or regulatory guidelines and standards for devices such as medical ultrasound equipment can ensure the safety and effectiveness of these products. For example, the FDA developed a regulatory standard for ultrasound therapy products[4] after the need had been established for reliable calibration and performance of this equipment.[14] This standard requires that ultrasound therapy products manufactured or marketed in the United States be adequately calibrated so that a prescribed amount of ultrasound energy can be delivered to the patient.

The development of standards and guidelines can also be used to encourage a consensus among the manufacturers and users concerning the specifications and performance of such devices. An example is the development of the voluntary "Safety Standard for Diagnostic Ultrasound Equipment" developed cooperatively by the AIUM and the NEMA partially in response to the FDA Notice of Intent[7] to examine the need for regulatory standards in diagnostic ultrasound. This standard fills the industry's need for standardized and accepted methods of measuring and reporting exposure information for diagnostic ultrasound equipment.

The standard also serves as a good example in which voluntary and regulatory efforts can be complementary to one another. Under the reporting requirements of the Radiation Control for Health and Safety Act of 1968 (PL 90–602) and the Medical Device Amendments of 1976 to the Food, Drug and Cosmetic Act, manufacturers are required to report patient exposures and other performance-related information. To assist a manufacturer in providing this information, a reporting guide developed by FDA was prepared to be consistent, where practicable, with the definitions used in the AIUM/NEMA standard. The information obtained from these reports serves as important function in monitoring any trends in the patient exposure levels associated with such equipment. Thus far, information obtained from these reports have shown that ultrasound emissions vary widely for different equipment designed to perform the same function.[15]

John C. Villforth
Director, National Center for Devices and
Radiological Health
Food and Drug Administration
Rockville, Maryland

●

In any developing field of activity, pressures build up for the adoption of standards and guidelines as techniques begin to mature. There are four main reasons for this. Firstly, measurements have to be made to ensure that proper account is taken of safety, often by balancing benefit against risk. Secondly, equipment performance has to be expressed in ways which allow results obtained by different investigators working in different laboratories to be compared and transferred. Third, manufacturers and users find it helpful to have design and performance specifications. Finally, agencies exist whose business it is to see to it that uniform standards are applied in the applications of methods which are either inherently hazardous, or are in widespread use, or both.

In the medical applications of ultrasound, the safety of three groups of individuals needs to be considered. These are the general public, the health workers, and the patients being investigated or treated. Existing guidelines do not seem to distinguish between these groups. This may be partly because the field is rather new, and partly because so little is known about real ultrasonic hazards. The present approach is to try to avoid all exposures to intensities above some particular levels, such as 100 mW/cm^2 SPTA and 3 W/cm^2 SATP at megahertz frequencies. These levels are not arbitrarily chosen, but are based on careful review of the existing evidence on ultrasonic bioeffects. Two main difficulties arise, however, as the results of this approach. Firstly, there seems to be an impression, at least in the minds of the relatively ill-informed, that exposures above the recommended levels are necessarily dangerous, and that lower exposures are certain to be safe. Secondly, no recognition is given to the principle that medical practitioners should not be constrained by regulations about exposure when deciding on the optimal benefit-risk compromises for any individual patient. (This principle is well accepted in diagnostic radiology, where there is no limit to the ionising radiation dose which can be administered to a patient provided that the medical practitioner is satisfied that the additional information that is obtained justifies the additional hazard.) Since resolution in diagnostic ultrasonic imaging is ultimately limited by the signal-to-noise ratio, it might be worth developing ultrasonic machines operating at much higher intensities than are "allowed" by the existing recommendations.

Standardization of diagnostic equipment performance also involves the specification of the image-forming process. The value of this in contributing toward the achievement of uniform image quality is uncontroversial. Writing standards for the image-forming process is much more difficult, however, than exposure and dose standardization, but it is beyond the scope of this volume.

In summary, it must be concluded that standards are useful. They should not be allowed, however, to limit innovation and progress. Moreover, in a rapidly developing field like medical ultrasonics, the formulation and enforcement of standards, particularly those of transient relevance, should not be allowed to consume more than a reasonable share of the available resources.

P.N.T. Wells, D.Sc.
Chief Physicist
Department of Medical Physics
Bristol General Hospital
Bristol, England

●

We trust that the above statements may be of interest to our colleagues and to all those who might be involved in formulating regulations and guidelines for the medical use of ultrasound. We thank all of the contributors for the thoughtful responses that they have so graciously provided.

REFERENCES

1. 100 Millimeter Test Object, Including Standard Procedure for its Use. American Institute of Ultrasound in Medicine, Bethesda, MD, 1974
2. Standard Specification of Echoscope Sensitivity and Noise Level, Including Recommended Practice for Such Measurements. American Institute of Ultrasound in Medicine, Bethesda, MD, 1979
3. Recommended Nomenclature: Physics and Engineering. American Institute of Ultrasound in Medicine, Bethesda, MD, 1980
4. Ultrasonic therapy products. Radiation safety performance standards. Fed Reg 43(34):7166, 1978
5. Ultrasound therapy device regulations. Can Gazette (Part II) 115(8):1121, 1981
6. Safety code 23. Guidelines for the Safe Use of Ultrasound, Part 1. Medical and Paramedical applications. Report 80-EHD-59. Environmental Health Directorate, Health Protection Branch, Ottawa, Canada, 1981

7. Diagnostic ultrasound equipment. Notice of intent to propose rules and develop recommendations. Fed Reg 44(31):9542, 1979

8. American Institute of Ultrasound in Medicine/National Electrical Manufacturers Association Safety Standard for Diagnostic Ultrasound Equipment. National Electrical Manufacturers Association Publication UL1-1981. Also published as Supplement to J Ultrasound Med, suppl., 2(4): S1, 1983

9. American Institute of Ultrasound in Medicine Commendation of Manufacturers. J Ultrasound Med 2:R6–7, 1983

10. Safety Considerations for Diagnostic Ultrasound. American Institute of Ultrasound in Medicine, Bethesda, MD, 1984

11. Biological Effects of Ultrasound: Mechanisms and Clinical Implications. National Council of Radiation Protection and Measurements. NCRP Report No. 74. NCRP Publications. Bethesda, MD, 1983

12. Environmental Health Criteria 22: Ultrasound. World Health Organization, Geneva, Switzerland, 1982

13. Hill CR, ter Haar G: Ultrasound. In Suess MJ (ed): Nonionizing Radiation Protection. World Health Organization, Regional Office for Europe, Copenhagen, 1982

14. Stewart HF, Harris GR, Herman BA, et al: Survey of Use and Performance of Ultrasonic Therapy Equipment in Pinellas County, Florida. Department of Health, Education and Welfare Publication (FDA) 73–8039, US Government Printing Office, Washington, DC, 1973

15. Stewart H: Outputs Levels from Commercial Diagnostic Ultrasound Equipment. Proceedings 28th Annual Convention of the American Institute of Ultrasound in Medicine, New York, October 18–21, 1983. J Ultrasound Med, suppl., 2(10):39, 1983

Appendix: Exposure Parameters for Diagnostic Equipment

WESLEY L. NYBORG

It is widely agreed (see Chapter 14) that output data for diagnostic ultrasound equipment should be made available to users. The American Institute of Ultrasound in Medicine—National Electrical Manufacturers Association (AIUM-NEMA) Standard lists and defines a number of parameters which are recommended for characterizing the output field. These well-defined parameters are referred to by the Food and Drug Administration (FDA) in its regulatory activities, and also by the AIUM in its Commendation process.

To receive the AIUM Commendation for an item of equipment, a manufacturer is required to provide technical data for the equipment, specifically on those items that are listed in Table 2.5. These must be made conveniently available to any interested persons so that the information can be used in making decisions on equipment or procedures. Some representative data obtained from recipients of the AIUM Commendation are given in Table A.1. For each of five classes of equipment, typical spatial-peak temporal-average (SPTA) and spatial-peak pulse-average (SPPA) intensities are shown; these quantities are defined in Chapter 2. The data in each row are for a specific transducer attached to and driven by a specific system; that is, each row is for a specific transducer-system (T/S) combination. Thus data are shown on four different T/S combinations for linear scanners, on three for manual B-scanners, on two each for pulsed and continuous Doppler equipment and on two for sector scanners. "Absolute maximum" values* are given for all intensities, as required for the AIUM Commendation; "typical" values are usually given also. It should be noticed that in Table A.1 SPTA values are given in milliwatts per square centimeter, while SPPA values are in watts per square centimeter.

* Absolute maximum values are values which the manufacturer states will not be exceeded. See Reference 8 of Chapter 14.

Of the equipment categories, it is the (sequential) linear arrays for which the intensities are usually lowest. The (absolute maximum) SPTA values range from 0.022 to 0.23 mW/cm² for the four T/S combinations whose specifications are listed in Table A.1. Comparison of entries shows that the SPPA intensities are more than 10,000 times the SPTA values. This is understandable since (1) the ultrasound is "on" during only a small fraction (e.g., 0.001) of the time and (2) the ultrasound beam is continuously swept through a range of positions so that it passes through a given point during only a fraction (e.g., 0.1) of the scan period.

From Table A.1 it is seen that for manual B-scanners the SPTA intensities (absolute maximum) for three T/S combinations vary from 35 to 116 mW/cm² while SPPA values vary from 96 to 168 W/cm². For these devices the SPTA intensity (by AIUM requirement) is defined for the transducer held in

TABLE A.1   Intensities for selected transducer-system (T/S) combinations[a]

Equipment Category	SPTA (mW/cm²)		SPPA (W/cm²)	
	Typ.	Abs. Max.	Typ.	Abs. max.
Linear array	—	0.033	—	0.40
	—	0.022	—	0.52
	—	0.21	—	3.1
	—	0.23	—	7.8
B-scanner	23	35	64	96
	38	57	61	91
	78	116	112	168
Pulsed Doppler	67	120	3	18
	80	155	3.6	22
Continuous Doppler	295	440	—	—
	335	500	—	—
	SPTA (mW/cm²)			SPPA (W/cm²)
Sector scanners	90°	45°	Freeze	
Abs. max. (typ.)	1.7 (0.8)	3.3 (1.6)	30 (13)	50 (21)
	2.5 (0.8)	5.0 (1.6)	54 (16)	150 (49)

[a] Data are from recipients of the AIUM Manufacturer's Commendation. *Abbreviations:* abs. max., absolute maximum, typ., typical.

a fixed position; during scanning it would have a lower value since the ultrasound beam then traverses a given location only a fraction of the time.

For pulsed-Doppler devices we see from Table A.1 that SPTA values tend to be somewhat higher, and SPPA values lower, than for manual B-scanners; this reflects the fact that for these devices the ultrasound is "on" for a larger fraction of the time. The SPPA data apply to equipment for which the operator is able to adjust the SPPA intensity up to the "absolute maximum" values shown; the "typical" values are for the different possible settings.

For continuous-Doppler equipment of the type represented in Table A.1 the SPTA intensity is higher than for other categories of diagnostic equipment. This equipment is designed to monitor blood flow in, for example, the femoral or carotid artery. The relatively high intensities are used so that ultrasound scattered from blood cells can be received.

The data for sector scanners given in Table A.1 show directly how the SPTA intensity (which is the temporal average at a fixed point) varies with the scanning mode. Thus for one of the T/S combinations the absolute maximum SPTA intensity is 1.7 mW/cm² in the 90° scanning mode, 3.3 mW/cm² in the 45° mode, and 30 mW/cm² in the freeze mode. On the other hand, the corresponding SPPA intensity is the same, 50 W/cm², in all modes.

As shown by published surveys, (see, e.g., references 11–13 of Chapter 14) there is much variation in output intensities of commercial equipment, with some generating much higher levels than those shown in Table A.1. Data for specific instruments can be obtained directly from published technical material for those firms who have received the AIUM Manufacturer's Commendation; those with Commendations for 1984 are: ADR Ultrasound, Technicare Ultrasound, Philips Ultrasound, General Electric Medical Systems, Diasonics, Inc., and Corometrics Medical Systems.

Index

Page numbers followed by *t* denote tables.